A MIND APART

A MIND APART

Poems of Melancholy, Madness, and Addiction

Edited by

MARK S. BAUER

OXFORD
UNIVERSITY PRESS
2009

OXFORD
UNIVERSITY PRESS

Oxford University Press, Inc., publishes works that further
Oxford University's objective of excellence
in research, scholarship, and education.

Oxford   New York
Auckland   Cape Town   Dar es Salaam   Hong Kong   Karachi
Kuala Lumpur   Madrid   Melbourne   Mexico City   Nairobi
New Delhi   Shanghai   Taipei   Toronto

With offices in
Argentina   Austria   Brazil   Chile   Czech Republic   France   Greece
Guatemala   Hungary   Italy   Japan   Poland   Portugal   Singapore
South Korea   Switzerland   Thailand   Turkey   Ukraine   Vietnam

Published by Oxford University Press, Inc.
198 Madison Avenue, New York, NY 10016

www.oup.com

Oxford is a registered trademark of Oxford University Press

Library of Congress Cataloging-in-Publication Data
A mind apart: poems of melancholy, madness and addiction/
edited by Mark S. Bauer.
p.   cm.
Includes bibliographical references and index.
ISBN 978-0-19-533640-5 (cloth) — ISBN 978-0-19-533641-2 (pbk.)
1. Melancholy—Poetry.   2. Mental illness—Poetry.   3. English poetry.
4. American poetry.   5. Substance abuse—Poetry.   6. Manic-depressive illness—Poetry.
7. Manic-depressive persons—Poetry.   8. Melancholy in literature.
9. Mental illness in literature.   I. Bauer, Mark S.
PR1195.M36M56 2008
821.009
2008012162

1 3 5 7 9 8 6 4 2

Printed in the United States of America
on acid-free paper

De profundis clamavi . . .
Out of the depths I cried . . .

—Psalm 130

*James once noted that Darwin gave up reading poetry
for years and then, finding it impossible to pick it up again,
wished that he had not let it go. James himself read
poetry—actively read poetry—all his life.*

—R. D. Richardson, *William James: In the
Maelstrom of American Modernism*

To my families

CONTENTS

PREFACE

In the spring of 2005 our local chapter of the Depression and Bipolar Support Alliance asked me to give a reading of poetry at the juncture of National Poetry Month and National Mental Health Month. A good idea, I thought. Who could not help but be moved by Gerard Manley Hopkins's "terrible sonnets" and by Robert Lowell's poetry on his manic-depressive illness and consequent hospitalizations? Who would not be intrigued, challenged—even frightened or repulsed—by the harsh lines of Anne Sexton or Franz Wright describing their difficulties and treatments? Such poems, read as poems, convey far more than one would take away by reading them as clinical specimens pinned under glass, or by sanctifying them as one might from a literal reading of Emily Dickinson's line "Much Madness is divinest Sense." To appreciate the variety and depth of such poetry is to be fundamentally touched by the poets' experience, and to recognize these experiences as integral aspects of the human condition in all its beauty and pain. The organizers of the reading also knew that to hear such poetry is, ultimately, a destigmatizing and hope-engendering experience.

I figured that it would be easy enough to prepare the reading: I'd just drop by the university library on my way home from the hospital some afternoon, pick a couple of relevant anthologies off the shelf, and go home and choose an hour's worth of poems to read. I learned, however, that such anthologies did not exist. Certainly there were a few "outsider" anthologies, typically the work of "patient" or "survivor" poets—but these were arguably more clinical or political than literary in orientation.

But there simply were no English-language anthologies of the poetry of . . . *what*? Of madness? Of melancholy? Of mental illness? Of neurasthenia or hysteria or bipolar disorder or schizophrenia or post-traumatic stress or alcoholism? Or of something altogether different? Where to begin? How to frame the issue? How to select the poems?

Where one begins determines in large part where one will end up (and this is just as true in science as in literary endeavors). Among the many possible beginnings, it seemed reasonable to gather poems that had been published somewhere—in journal, book, or broadside—that were in some way relevant to current conceptions of "mental illness" (in psychiatric terms) or "madness" (in cultural criticism terms). Thus, twenty-first-century clinical and critical vantage points would serve as a trawling net to collect poems for the reading. And as we shall see, nets being nets, this one turned out to be more air than fiber.

The introduction that follows describes how this trawling net was woven from both clinical and critical strands, and how the weaving affected the catch that was eventually scooped aboard. Thus, while the poems certainly stand on their own, the introduction will be of interest to the reader who is curious about the concepts of "madness" or "mental illness," how these concepts informed the choice of poems, how they can inform their reading, and how each of these two constructs leaves us far short of being able to fully comprehend such conditions.

The reader will quickly note that the selection is limited to poems written in English. Accordingly, the clinical-critical discussion in the introduction can safely be applied no further than certain Anglophone cultures. The discussion must start somewhere. Homer, Job, Li Ch'ing-chao, Tasso, Baudelaire, Lermontov, Pavese, and myriad others await the more erudite.

Before beginning, there are some debts to gratefully acknowledge. A variety of colleagues from diverse backgrounds and perspectives helped me to test out the concepts and the logic of the introduction and flesh out the implications of this project. Chief among these is my wife and most careful and caring critic, Beth Wietelmann Bauer. In addition, C. Andrew Buck, Giselle Corre, Thomas D'Evelyn, Robert Howard, April Peters, Paul Pirraglia, and Jeff Poland provided extensive commentary. Nicki Sahlin, former executive director of the Rhode Island chapter of the National Alliance for the Mentally Ill, provided cogent discussion around these issues as well. Very special thanks go to Donna Howard, executive director of the Depression and Bipolar Support Alliance, East Bay chapter, whose invitation stimulated this project.

Alongside every scholar stands a savvy librarian. I am particularly indebted to Rosemary Cullen and the staff of the John Hay Library of Brown University for their expert and patient help, and for access to rare manuscripts and other resources otherwise unavailable. At Oxford University Press, Shannon McLachlan and Christina Gibson, and their anonymous reviewers, have been of great help in bringing this manuscript into final form.

I also appreciate support from Brown University's Salomon Research Fund for what must have seemed to them a high-risk project: a psychiatrist embarking on a literary project and promising payoff both for clinical and for critical fields. Additionally, I am grateful for a Brown University Karen T. Romer Undergraduate Teaching and Research Award supporting Esme Cullen, whose research on the lives of the poets included here was invaluable.

I wish also to acknowledge my ongoing debt to the U.S. Department of Veterans Affairs where, I recently realized, I seem to have spent the majority of my psychiatric clinical career caring for veterans and their families, teaching, conducting research, and from time to time doing health care administration. The VA, first the Providence VA Medical Center and now the VA Boston Healthcare System, has provided a clinical home for me and an intellectual stimulus to much of my work, including this project.

Finally, I am grateful to Christina Moniz for her assistance with manuscript preparation. As with our many other projects, she has been efficient and unfailingly accurate.

Mark S. Bauer, M.D.
Brockton, Massachusetts
December 2007

A MIND APART

INTRODUCTION

1. Setting the Stage

The argument. Every anthology makes an argument. Few anthologists, however, will come out and tell you what it is. Take, for instance, the anthologist's selection of individual poems and poets. The argument, unstated, is, "This or that poet is worth including, is canonical," and so forth. That this is indeed the stuff of argument becomes clear when the point-counterpoint reviews that inevitably follow the publication of noteworthy anthologies begin to appear.

Even more subtly, the structure that an anthologist gives an anthology also makes an argument. What qualifies, for example, as "Victorian" or "feminist" or "postmodern" poetry? Is it a time, a theme, a habit of thought, a shadow of influence? Even chronological boundaries are not as evident as they seem at first: I might argue, for instance, that nineteenth-century poetry ended not in 1900 but with a pistol's crack in June 1914. Still greater challenges attend the making of an anthology of poetry related in some way to "mental illness" or "madness." How one defines these terms is of more than purely literary import, as we shall see below.

It is not a new idea that such states may be related to poetic creativity. In the fourth century BCE, Theophrastus asked in "Problem XXX, I": "Why is it that all those who have become eminent in philosophy, politics, poetry, or the arts are clearly melancholics . . .?" This query has followed us down millennia, and a number of commonsense questions follow from it. Was Christopher Smart mad or sane when he wrote the sprawling verses to his cat, Jeoffry? Are John Clare's "I Am" poems the product of melancholia? Did Robert Lowell's flagrant manic episodes help or hurt his poetry? Could Sylvia Plath or Anne Sexton have written such moving poetry without suffering depression so brutal that it led them to suicide?

These are indeed commonsense questions. However, they are not the most informative questions to ask. They introduce a subtle reductionism, whether approached from the clinical perspective or from the perspective of cultural and literary criticism. Each assumes that one knows what "mental illness" or "madness" is. And such subtle reductionism creeps in regardless of whether we think it is chemistry or culture that causes the phenomena, and regardless of whether we think affected individuals should be medicated or looked to for platonic Truth. Rather, the more fundamental questions that confront us are: What is this "thing" that some call "mental illness" and others call "madness"? How is it some describable other thing? How does such a dichotomized approach help us, and how does it get in the way of our perception?

Whatever the label, these phenomena have somehow to do with the wholesale loosening of conventions of thought, perception, and behavior; destructive inner torment or emptiness; or effects of habitual use of, or acute deprivation of, external substances. *Somehow* to do with these—but how, exactly? Honoring this complexity, and aware of the tentativeness of our understanding, we will speak of mental illnesses, or madness, as *constructs*. This term recognizes that while these experiences exist, they are only imprecisely definable. We who conceptualize them impose—construct—around them knowable, utilitarian, but constantly evolving and always somewhat wrong definitions so that we can communicate about them. As Corinne Saunders and Jane Macnaughton put it in their volume of essays on the occasion of the founding of the University of Durham's innovative Centre for Arts and Humanities in Health and Medicine, the process of truly understanding such conditions is best conceived of as "a dialogue between medicine and literature."[1]

So, with attention to both clinical and critical aspects, how can these constructs be understood? To be specific: What will be the bounds of this anthology?

Categories in current psychiatric research and practice. The major clinical and scientific schemata for psychiatric diagnosis in use today are the American Psychiatric Association's *Diagnostic and Statistical Manual* (*DSM*, currently in its fourth edition) and the *International Classification of Diseases* (*ICD*, currently in its tenth edition). These systems present a series of diagnostic categories that are distinguished from one another, and from normal mental function and behavior, based on the presence of certain behaviors and reported symptoms.

They purport only to describe and not invoke underlying mechanisms, either psychosocial or biologic (though this claim is open to question). The categories are designed to be mutually exclusive, though individuals often have more than one diagnosis. (A curious sidelight: Only individuals can "officially" be ill—not couples, and certainly not entire cultures or societies or nations.)

This kind of *categorical* thinking leads to a view of mental illness that says either you have X or you do not; either you have Y or you do not; moreover, X and Y are distinct disorders. While these systems do not explicitly state that you are either "sick" or you are "normal," the implication is there: Either you meet criteria for a disorder or you do not.

Cultural criticism and psychiatric diagnosis. Psychiatry, like most fields, tends not to self-examine and prefers not to question the assumptions that underlie the data and the hypotheses from which the data derive. Cultural critics and historians of science have been more than happy to fill this gap.

Perhaps the most influential critique of the underpinnings of psychiatry was Michel Foucault's *Madness and Civilization* in the early 1960s. Foucault's main point was that mental illnesses are not invariant phenomena waiting to be discovered and characterized like geological strata or insects, but rather are social fabrications. Though fatally flawed as traditional history, Foucault's work effectively highlighted the social aspects of psychiatric diagnosis and treatment. The most radical use of this theme was that of the proponents of "antipsychiatry," such as R. D. Laing and Thomas Szaz. This movement, prominent in the 1960s and 1970s, proposed that mental illness diagnoses themselves were societal labels imposed on gullible victims for the gain of a select elite.

These decades were a time not only of substantial sociopolitical turmoil but also of tremendous progress in the biological sciences. For psychiatry it was the time of widespread introduction of lithium, antidepressants, and antipsychotics, which revolutionized the treatment of many mental illnesses. It was, not surprisingly, a time that foregrounded the split between cultural and clinical (and increasingly biological) views of these phenomena. However, as Roy Porter and other historians of psychiatry have pointed out, this tension between sociocultural and biomedical explanations for mental illness can be traced back in Western culture at least to the Greeks.

In current times, most cultural critics and historians of psychiatry accept that mental illnesses are not simply social constructions. However, they focus primarily on the social and cultural factors that shape our understanding of these constructs with, at times, a curious lack of attention to the phenomena themselves that undoubtedly shape the sociocultural response. Example: If a person with mania is doused, exorcised, punished, psychoanalyzed, medicated, electroshocked, and so forth, what role might the person's impulsive, grandiose, labile, hypersexual, demanding, ebullient, overconfident, short-tempered behavior itself have had to do with society's response? And why do these behaviors themselves show up in so many cultural contexts across the centuries looking so very similar?

Thus, reasoned cultural criticism of psychiatry serves a valuable function, elucidating the many assumptions and sources of influence that contribute to clinical and scientific psychiatry as practiced today. However, in isolation from clinical science, cultural criticism cannot provide a comprehensive understanding of mental illness, but only a critique of the social aspects of disorders and their diagnosis.

In a series of classic articles in the turbulent 1970s, George Engel proposed that mental illnesses—and in fact *all* illnesses, including even acute events like heart attacks—have not only biological but also psychological and social determinants. Though aimed primarily at those seduced by the remarkable advances in biological science into neglecting psychological and social aspects of illness, Engel's criticism could have been applied as well to his contemporary antipsychiatrists and cultural critics who would limit their attention to the social components of illness, particularly mental disorders. Now, thirty years later, we can extend Engel's "biopsychosocial model": *Comprehensive understanding of mental illness requires consideration of the biological, psychological, and social factors that produce these phenomena, in conjunction with consideration of the social and cultural filters that affect how we perceive, conceptualize, investigate, and respond to them.* In order to better appreciate these poems, we will work from this expanded biopsychosocial perspective, and we will begin by reconsidering one of the currently most powerful paradigms in psychiatry, that of categorical diagnosis. We will then suggest an alternative method of understanding these constructs in light of the poetry at hand.

A dimensional understanding of human behavior. Lurking, often unrecognized, at the edges of the categorical schemata outlined above, are milder, or "subsyndromal," forms of the disorders that the diagnostic systems delineate. For instance, major depressive disorder has been firmly established as a diagnosis for several decades, as has its milder, more chronic cousin, dysthymia; even milder, subsyndromal depression has been well demonstrated in community surveys as well. Manic-depressive disorder (now known by its less accurate name, "bipolar disorder") includes type I (with severe mania) and type II (with less severe hypomania); cyclothymia delineates an even milder version, while lesser forms of mood excursions, "bipolar III, IV, V . . . ," are the subject of ongoing research. Even schizophrenia, so distinct in full form, has milder related forms that are considered personality disorders, yet are linked to schizophrenia by a number of biological and familial characteristics. Evidence is also accumulating that indicates that boundaries between diagnoses are less distinct than a categorical system would seem to imply. For instance, modern genetic evidence suggests bipolar disorder and schizophrenia, considered quite distinct since the days of Emil Kraepelin, the "father" of modern psychiatric diagnosis, may also be part of a single spectrum. The case is similar for the boundary between depressive and anxiety disorders.

These and numerous other examples indicate clearly that the categorical approach to mental illness and normalcy is frayed around the edges. Mental illnesses are thus more accurately conceived of not as categories but as *dimensions*—continua or spectra without clear separation from normalcy, and with less separation from each other than we like to think. A useful analogy is provided by high blood pressure (or, by its categorical name, hypertension). Clearly, blood pressure is a dimensional continuum, not an either/or category into which some people fall and others don't. Rather, for some people in some situations, blood pressure higher than a certain level causes problems; in other people, the same level may not. *On average*, a particular level of blood pressure *usually* causes problems. At some levels it *always* does. Thus there is precedent for conceptualizing these constructs as dimensions that are not so readily separable from normalcy, except in their more severe forms.

An intriguing side issue is why clinical medicine and science have not recognized this dimensionality as the major diagnostic paradigm. There are historical and philosophical reasons: Psychiatry and to a degree psychology see themselves as subdisciplines of medicine, and medicine has diagnoses. There are also heuristic reasons: It is more difficult to study dimensions than to study yes/no categories. And clinically, it is more difficult to decide whom to treat if the problem is a dimension and not a category of ill/well. Finally, there is an economic component: How do you bill for treating something that is not a disease, something that may be an extreme of a continuum—and how do the payers know when to stop paying?

Genetics, temperament, and dimensional views of mental illness. Genetics, that most categorical of sciences, in actuality leads us even further in the dimensional direction. It once was thought that each mental illness was transmitted by a single gene on a chromosome: Get the gene from one or both of your parents and you develop a disorder;

don't get the gene, and you don't develop a disorder. However, the actual data are more complicated—and more biopsychosocial. Even identical twins, who have exactly the same genetic material, "match" for manic-depressive illness or schizophrenia only about 40–70 percent of the time. These "concordance" rates are even lower for depression. So development, either in utero or in the wider world, must play a role. Clearly, genetics is not destiny.

Behavioral genetics points toward a further provocative possibility: That it is not the disorders themselves that are passed on genetically, but rather *temperaments* that predispose one to eventually develop a mental illness. *Temperament* can be defined as a tendency from infancy to *perceive* and *respond to* the world in a particular manner. For instance, some infants appear to be born with a tendency to avoid novelty, and others to seek it out. Some respond to new objects, novel situations, or strangers with fear and avoidance while others are not bothered, and some even appear eager to explore. Not surprisingly, temperaments are also dimensions, not categories. Moreover, every one of us manifests a variety of temperamental characteristics from birth: Temperament research has left our revered *tabula rasa* shattered in the dustbin.

Further, some of these genetically inherited temperaments are associated with the development of *DSM*-defined disorders; for example, a temperament measured as "behavioral inhibition" in young children is strongly associated with the later development of anxiety disorders. But just as genetics is not destiny, neither is temperament: The eventual development of anxiety disorders depends on temperament-environment interactions, and the same appears to be true for the recurrent "bad" behaviors of antisocial personalities as well—again underscoring the need for a biopsychosocial understanding of these constructs.

So: What is passed on through generations is not likely mental illness per se, but rather the tendency to see and respond to the world in a particular way. The probability of developing what we now call a mental illness will therefore be a product of the interaction of environment with such tendencies. Not surprisingly, this is expressed as a spectrum or dimension of severity.

Thus, based on the scientific evidence alone—even without considering its cultural underpinnings—there appears no clear border between this aggregate of mental disorders and normalcy. These constructs are dimensional: there is no clear *Other*.

Nonetheless, severe and disabling mental illnesses *do* exist—as anyone who has spent significant time with those who suffer from such states can attest. How to resolve this paradox? And, for clinicians (and insurers and administrators and employers and teachers and parents and spouses and others), how to understand and how to intervene? Astute clinicians, consciously or unconsciously, apply a "fuzzy set" approach to diagnosis: While classic instances are clear and severe, when one approaches the borders of another category, the diagnosis becomes murky and the treatment path becomes less certain. Similarly, as one approaches the border with normalcy, the pathology becomes less evident, as do the disability and the attendant imperative to treat.

A dimensional understanding of the poems. Therefore, because it is impossible to delineate firm categories of "mad" and "sane," "mentally ill" and "normal," our reading of these poems must move beyond attributing their content to a particular pathological state—and must also move beyond spending time disproving this assertion. Instead, understanding these constructs as *tendencies*—tendencies to perceive and to respond to one's world in particular ways—opens us up to a broader reading of the poems (and a broader reading of what we have come to call mental illness or madness).

What are the implications of this for reading these poems? These poets—and all of us—are born with tendencies, conferred genetically. Certainly, social and cultural factors impact how these tendencies will be expressed (while other social and cultural factors determine how society will respond to the resultant behavior). Since these tendencies are genetically transmitted, they should be highly conserved over the relatively short time frame (for evolution) of seven centuries. Thus, we may then find patterns across poems that reflect these (dimensional) constructs, and identifying these patterns will enrich our understanding of the poems and the poets. Additionally, we would expect that these patterns, though identifiable, will be expressed in terms that conform to the poetic habits of each age, and to the life history and vision of the individual poet. The construct of "melancholy" provides perhaps the most striking example, and it is traced it out in some detail in the next section of this introduction.

Note, though, that none of this implies that a poet necessarily writes "about" melancholy or depression or hysteria or any other such construct. Considering only a poet's conscious intention in writing a particular poem has been justly out of favor for decades, and if it were possible to query a long-dead poet, or one not so long dead, or if we were to query any one of many still living in this age of modern diagnosis, "Were you writing about . . .?" many would scoff. On the other hand, close (or closed) reading of a poem as a hermetically sealed object, to which cultural factors and individual life history are of accidental relevance, provides quite limited comprehension. It is also terribly limiting to read these poems from the confines of current clinical diagnoses as has been frequently done in psychohistorical and psychoanalytic studies. Similarly, these poems cannot be fully understood as solely a function of their cultural context. Each of these filters will screen out important information and limit our appreciation of the poems.

Rather, we propose to read *across* poems and *across* epochs for commonalities. This approach is more closely akin to qualitative research methods that are increasingly used in clinical research to understand experiences from the patient's perspective and to reduce reliance on a priori hypotheses that the investigator brings to the investigation. Recall, however, that all critical and all scientific studies must start from some initial conditions, and ours, as we have openly confessed, is the trawling net of twenty-first-century clinical descriptions of various types of "mental illness" or "madness." Yes, the dimensional understanding of these conditions has left our net frayed around the edges—but the fraying itself will bring us a better catch.

Yet to focus solely on commonality would also be reductionistic. As John Z. Sadler has effectively pointed out in *Values and Psychiatric Diagnosis*, modern psychiatric assessment tends to suffer from "hyponarrativity," a lack of attention to the life in which the various symptoms are embedded. (George Engel would have concurred.) We thus will read these poems not only for commonality, which we expect given the net we have used, but also for difference. Such differences are to be anticipated given the breadth of epochs, sociocultural settings, life histories, and myriad other factors that characterize so wide a swath of poetry. Reading for difference between, say, Jane Kenyon's and Gerard Manley Hopkins's treatment of despondency, or Emily Dickinson's and Thomas Hoccleve's treatment of stigma, makes evident the variety and richness of the specific voices that carry these concerns. At the same time such differences also throw into even starker relief the commonalities that do endure across epochs, cultures, and individuals. Thus we read each poem as the product of an individual life lived in a specific sociocultural context, yet also as evidence of a common thread that links these diverse lives across epochs.

Recognizing both the commonalities and the differences among these poems also enhances our understanding of the underlying constructs. These we understand not primarily as illnesses (though in severe instances they are, in all senses, illnesses) and not primarily as some Other to be inspected from a distance. Rather we appreciate them as multi-faceted, multi-determined, somewhat mysterious, and in some regards ubiquitous dimensions of human experience.

2. Reading the Poems

Let us now turn to the poems themselves, and look in some detail at how such constructs—experienced as *patterns* within and across the poems—emerge across epochs, cultures, and individuals. While not all patterns will appear in all poems, we will focus on three patterns that stand out for their recurrent and striking appearance across these centuries: melancholy, madness, and "sweet melancholy."

Melancholy. The first such pattern, which we will call "melancholy," emerges in diverse poems across several centuries. The pattern points toward an underlying construct that has something to do with what has been called (in "fuzzy set" fashion) melancholia, desolation, despondency, despair, dysthymia, major depressive disorder, and the like.

Jane Kenyon's "Having it Out with Melancholy" reads like a veritable companion for the *DSM* entry for major depressive disorder. There is even a heritable component (whether nature or nurture), in this case from her mother, as it begins "in the nursery" when she finds her mother figuratively lying on top of her,

> pressing
> the bile of desolation into every pore.

Kenyon is anhedonic, unable to feel pleasure in anything: "everything under the sun and moon/made me sad," and hopeless: "We're here simply to wait for death." She takes to her bed, hoping to be so lucky that sleep will muffle the pain:

> Often I go to bed as soon after dinner
> as seems adult
> (I mean I try to wait for dark)
> in order to push away
> from the massive pain . . .

She is slow of thought and deed, without desire, virtually without life beyond vegetal subsistence:

> A piece of burned meat
> wears my clothes, speaks
> in my voice,
> dispatches obligations
> haltingly, or not at all.

Even her dog is more fully functional, and keeps her from suicide:

> The dog searches until he finds me
> upstairs, lies down with a clatter
> of elbows, puts his head on my foot.
>
> Sometimes the sound of his breathing
> saves my life . . .

She is overcome by a distinct feeling, different from sadness; then, mysteriously, this "pain stops/abruptly" with medication treatment. She puzzles over the foreignness of this state, as antidepressants begin to take effect:

> With the wonder
> and bitterness of someone pardoned
> for a crime she did not commit.

Her social isolation and withdrawal gradually abate: "I come back to marriage and friends." She returns to the enjoyment of everyday things around her, "to pink fringed hollyhocks." She takes up again, finally, her life's work, coming back "to my desk, books, and chair."

Jim Harrison, in "Sequence I," never speaks of depression or melancholy, yet clearly portrays the black bile of melancholics who have

> black roots in their brains
> around which vessels clot.

These eat away at life:

> The roots feed on the brain until the brain is all
>   root—now the brain is gray
> and suffocates in its own folds.

Sylvia Plath's "Street Song" conveys the unique and inarticulable pain, and resultant isolation, with a deft image:

> my each mangled nerve-end
> Trills its hurt out
> Above pitch of pedestrian ear.

In Edna St. Vincent Millay's "Sorrow," her psychic pain stands in contrast to physical pain:

> People twist and scream in pain,—
> Dawn will find them still again

Her psychic pain, though, is unforgiving and relentless:

> This has neither wax nor wane,
>   Neither stop nor start.

She describes in briefest strokes the mental and physical slowing and the social isolation that characterize this state:

> People dress and go to town;
>   I sit in my chair.
> All my thoughts are slow and brown:
> Standing up or sitting down
> Little matters, or what gown
>   Or what shoes I wear

—all rendered more vivid by the relentlessness of the stretched out vowel sounds in "town," "slow," "brown," "down," and "gown." Dylan Thomas's "Out of the Sighs" clearly differentiates this state from grief and loss (even within the poem's context of grief and loss):

> Out of the sighs a little comes,
> But not of grief, for I have knocked down that
> Before the agony . . .

Still earlier in the twentieth century, Edward Thomas's "Melancholy" conveys the vague sense of incompletion, of emptiness, and of hopelessness that the feeling can ever be resolved:

> What I desired I knew not, but whate'er my choice
> Vain it must be, I knew.

There are also twentieth century poems, both from the current age of modern diagnosis and earlier, that stand at further remove from explicit description of depression, melancholy, or the like. Among the most powerful of such poems is Donald Justice's "The Man Closing

Up." Manifestly the simple scene of a lighthouse keeper at dusk, the poem opens, simply:

> Like a deserted beach,
> The man closing up.

The man is not *on* a deserted beach; the man *is* a deserted beach, desert-ed, desiccated. We learn from Justice's spare lines, almost in passing, that

> He has no hunger
> For anything,

and later

> He would make his bed,
> If he could sleep on it.
>
> He would make his bed with white sheets
> And disappear into the white.

Time crawls by. In his isolation he gropes for

> A simple word,
> . . .
> He wants to keep the light going,
> If he can.

The psychoanalyst and critic Julia Kristeva has suggested that clinical depression is intimately related to the inability to use language to structure one's world and one's experience of self. The lighthouse keeper is left wordless in his melancholy; the poem ends:

> the man closing up
> Does not say the word.

In earlier poems this sense of lack, of Edward Thomas's "what I desired I knew not," is occasionally named, even in familiar terms. As long ago as the early 1700s Anne Finch in her "The Spleen: A Pindaric Poem" refers to "our deprest and pond'rous Frame," while in the early nineteenth century we find Thomas Bayly speaking of "the depression already too strong" in his poem of recovery that begins "I welcome thee back again, Spirit of Song!"

More often the pattern will take a name more familiar to the epoch, as in Samuel Taylor Coleridge's "Dejection: An Ode" or John Keats's "Ode on Melancholy," or as in Ernest Dowson's "Spleen" later in the 1800s. This last poet also clearly differentiates his state from sadness:

> I was not sorrowful, I could not weep
> . . .
> I was not sorrowful, but only tired
> Of everything that ever I desired.

The pattern in Coleridge's "Dejection: An Ode" makes the same differentiation between sadness or grief and the melancholic construct:

> A grief without a pang, void, dark, and drear,
> A stifled, drowsy, unimpassioned grief.

In a single line he provides as poignant and accurate a description as is found in any modern medical dictionary of the symptom currently called "anhedonia," the lack of ability to feel pleasure; he looks around at his bucolic surroundings, and the only response he can summon is "I see, not feel, how beautiful they are!"

In other nineteenth-century poems melancholy stands unnamed, yet potent. In the mid-1800s Emily Dickinson, the master of "telling it slant," fights against "The Cavalry of Woe" in #126. In #670 she describes for us that

> The Brain has Corridors—surpassing
> Material Place—
>
> Far safer, of a Midnight Meeting
> External Ghost
> Than its interior Confronting—
> That Cooler Host.

John Clare, roughly a contemporary of the Romantics, but possessing quite a different sensibility, tells us in his two "I Am" poems. In "Sonnet: I am" he is "dull and void" with his "soaring thoughts destroyed." In "I Am," nothing is left but inward-turning misery: "I am the self-consumer of my woes." His days and nights merge in unceasing, self-deprecating anhedonia:

> Into the nothingness of scorn and noise,—
> Into the living sea of waking dreams,

> Where there is neither sense of life or joys,
>   But the vast shipwreck of my lifes esteems.

He describes his puzzling emotional coldness even toward friends and family:

> Even the dearest, that I love the best
> Are strange—nay, rather stranger than the rest

—strikingly similar to Hayden Carruth's twentieth-century description of visiting hours in "The Asylum":

> Thus when our solemn inspectors come to stroll
> The shadeless halls, our wives and friends,
> We seldom mention how the winds
> Shriek in their mouths. Gradually we feel
> More natural, we try
> To sink like the silent leaves that slide and reel
> In anguish down the windy sky.

Not surprisingly, the melancholic pattern is frequently associated with loss, often loss of love. Emerging from the wide-ranging poetry of lost love, traces of this distinctive pattern, beyond simple sadness or grief, can be found at least as far back as Lady Mary Wroth's songs and sonnets in the 1600s; her loss turns all pleasure into its opposite:

> Light, leave thye light, fit for a lightsome soul;
> Darkness doth truly suit with me oppressed [Urania Sonnet XIX]

leaving her hopeless:

> The more shee strive, more deepe in Sand is prest
> Till she be lost: so am I in this kind
> Sunck, and devour'd, and swallow'd by unrest
>   [Amphilanthus Sonnet VI]

(Note, though, that many other distinctly non-melancholic patterns are also associated with lost love, as can be seen in Robert Herrick's seventeenth-century "Mad Maid's Song" and in the popular songs of the early nineteenth century, such as the "Crazy Jane" songs.)

The melancholic pattern also appears in the context of loss of a very different type—the silence of God. From Thomas Traherne in the

1600s we hear the familiar notes of desolation, withdrawal from one's social roles, and inability to work. He opens "Solitude":

> How desolate!
> Ah! how forlorn, how sadly did I stand
>   When in the field my woful State
>   I felt! Not all the Land,
>   Not all the Skies,
>   Tho Heven shin'd before mine Eys,
>   Could Comfort yield in any Field to me,
>   Nor could my Mind Contentment find or see.
>
>   Remov'd from Town,
>   From People, Churches, Feasts, and Holidays,
>   The Sword of State, the Mayor's Gown,
>   And all the Neighb'ring Boys;

Even his beloved Church cannot ease the pain:

> Th' External Rite,
> Altho the face be wondrous sweet and fair,
>   Can satiate my Appetit
>   No more than empty Air
>   Yield solid Food.

Similar desolation is found in several of George Herbert's seventeenth-century poems of religious struggle. In "Affliction (I)" he describes a life in which

> There was no month but May.
> But with my years sorrow did twist and grow.

Soon there is nothing left but sorrow:

> I scarce believed,
> Till grief did tell me roundly, that I lived.

And:

> My mirth and edge was lost: a blunted knife
>   Was of more use than I.

He loses weight and abandons his social life: "thin and lean, without a fence or friend." He is immobilized with indecision: "I could not go away, nor persevere," and self-condemning because of his uselessness:

> I read, and sigh, and wish I were a tree—
>   For sure, then, I should grow
> To fruit or shade; at least, some bird would trust
> Her household to me, and I should be just.

Again in "Affliction (IV)," he is but "a wonder tortur'd" whose

> thoughts are all a case of knives,
> Wounding my heart
> . . .
> Nothing their fury can control,
> While they do wound and prick my soul.

His faculties—his "attendants"—are

>   at strife
> Quitting their place
> Unto my face:
> Nothing performs the task of life.

He even reaches the point of suicide: "O help, my God! let not their plot / Kill them and me." The often-anthologized "The Collar" can be read in a similar vein, beginning with the title, the well-recognized pun on "choler" (the yellow bile of raving or rage). In commenting on "Affliction (IV)," poet, critic, and religion scholar Geoffrey Hill rightly maintains concurrent attention to both the spiritual and the melancholic aspects of Herbert's work: "He [Herbert] recognized the 'detail' for what it simultaneously is: a depressive sentiment, not an exclusive spiritual concept or a mystical hypothesis, however eloquent."[2]

Gerard Manley Hopkins wrote more recently, in the last half of the nineteenth century, and we have evidence from his correspondence and biographical information that he had periods of what we would now call clinical depression. In light of this evidence it is even easier to see the links between spiritual desolation and the melancholic construct that appear so poignantly in his "terrible sonnets."

The state is distinct, horrible, and far removed from normal sadness or grief:

> No worst, there is none. Pitched past pitch of grief,
> More pangs will, schooled at forepangs, wilder wring.

He finds himself on a precipice unknown to those who have not experienced it, hanging and perhaps ready to let go:

> O the mind, mind has mountains; cliffs of fall
> Frightful, sheer, no-man-fathomed. Hold them cheap
> May who ne'er hung there . . .

That this desolate state was not considered by such poets—or the majority of their readers—as other than spiritual in nature is not surprising. But a variety of sources indicate, in their very rejection of this link between spiritual desolation and melancholy, that such a link was indeed plausible and perhaps often considered. Consider, for instance, the eighteenth-century Quaker Samuel Bownas writing of such desolation:

> But finding ourselves very uneasy and in great trouble of mind, being under sorrow and heaviness, not rightly and coolly examining the reason, it is often mistaken to proceed from a material cause. And so outside means are sought for to relieve from this uneasiness; some by taking the bottle with their companions, others diverting themselves with sports or gaming, others taking medicines to help them against what they call melancholy.[3]

Thus, from the almost clinical recounting of Kenyon's "Having it Out with Melancholy" to the named and unnamed desolation of others in the age of modern diagnosis and far earlier, we find this melancholic construct portrayed in consistent patterns across the poems: sometimes physical, mental always, distinct and beyond sadness and grief, almost palpable. Often, but not always, this pattern is associated with loss, either loss of love or spiritual abandonment.

Because the melancholic pattern in these poems outstrips its link with loss, there must be a broader, deeper, and more persistent construct than can be accounted for simply by response to loss (Freud's "Mourning and Melancholia" notwithstanding). Whether refracted through the sensibilities of a poet like Kenyon, well familiar with modern clinical conceptions of mental illness, or through the pain of lost love in the seventeenth century, or through the spiritual vision of a nineteenth-century Jesuit priest, the core melancholic construct has *something* to do with emptiness and removal from persons and activities and things that make life worth living. Whatever its source, their perception and their response unite them: Out of the depths comes their cry.

Madness and reason. A second pattern that emerges among other poems across centuries is the opposition of madness to reason—specifically, that madness results from an abdication of reason in the face of drives and desires. Here we speak of "madness" generally as the wholesale loosening of conventions of thought, perception, and behavior. For almost clinical descriptions of this state we can turn to the popular songs of the early nineteenth century or the more modern vignette in Aimee Grunberger's "The Administration of Veterans."

Moving to earlier times, we find that madness is frequently counterposed to reason, which is represented not as some nonspecific source of self-control by a higher faculty but rather in the classical sense of logical, rational thought placed specifically in opposition to unruly passions that can lead to madness. To associate madness with the absence of control by reason may seem tautological; however, one need only look back to Plato's *Phaedrus* to see that such behavior has not always been considered a deficit of reason. For Plato, madness was "a nobler thing than sober sense."[4]

Shakespeare's Sonnet 129, perhaps the best known of such poems, tells us—in convoluted syntax, itself mimicking the twisted emotional knots that passion can engender—that lust, "past reason hunted," and "past reason hated" will "make the taker mad." A century later, Isaac Watts, battling a state that sounds like what modern diagnosticians would call mania, finds that

> In vain my reason gives
> The peaceful word, my spirit strives in vain
> To calm the tumult and command my thoughts.

But, alas, "The engine rules the man." He gives an intriguing proto-neurobiologic explanation:

> little restless atoms rise and reign
> Tyrants in sovereign uproar . . .

Despite his ride "thro' airy wilds unknown, with dreadful speed," he has a

> weary spirit, tost with tempests,
> Harass'd and broken

and longs to reach "the port of rest" when, finally,

> th'irregular springs of vital movement
> Ungovernable, return to sacred order,
> And pay their duties to the ruling mind.

Reason finally throttles back the engine.

The counterposing of rational, logical thought to madness is not only the province of the learned. Popular songs in the early nineteenth century echo this theme in their various descriptions of men and women gone mad. In the early twentieth century, the anonymous author of "Thoughts Suggested on a Thanksgiving Day Passed at the State Lunatic Asylum, Worcester, Mass., by a Patient" puts his faith in ordered, rational thought in the person of the physician since

> God has given in mercy thus
> To the discreet physician, to devise
> Such skilful schemes, and to them grants success

and also in the very routine of the asylum itself:

> That perfect neatness, which is wont to reign
> Within these walls. Here *order*, in its prime
> Presides, *system complete*, than which could be
> Nought perfect more; for all in concert move,
> With jarring seldom mix'd, confusion ne'er.

In our age of modern diagnosis, the opposition of rational thought to madness is less prominent. Neither psychoanalytic nor neuro-biological explanations of psychosis, nor postmodern critical thought, supports the notion that such a state can be "thought through" (though here in the age of cognitive therapy one wonders if the cortex is expected to rise again to attempt to subdue the limbic system). In fact, there are signs of disillusionment with reason as an antidote to madness quite a bit earlier, as Matthew Arnold's "Empedocles on

Etna" conveys. Empedocles is ready to leap into a volcano to his death, having lost his faith in reason; he has discarded his

> laurel bough!
> Scornful Apollo's ensign . . .

At the crater's rim he decries his loyalty to reason, despite having lived a rational life not subject to passions and desires:

> Slave of sense
> I have in no wise been; but slave of thought?
> And who can say: I have been always free,
> Lived ever in the light of my own soul?
> I cannot; I have lived in wrath and gloom.

And he jumps to a molten death.

"Sweet melancholy." The third pattern to examine in some detail is one of the more curious to emerge from these poems: "sweet melancholy." What, precisely, was so sweet about it? And is melancholy, in our age of modern diagnosis and treatment, still so sweet? One suspects that there is indeed some sweetness left: Otherwise there could be no quarrel that this condition, horrific and debilitating in full form, should at all costs be as comprehensively identified and vigorously treated as, say, cancer, heart disease, muscular dystrophy, or AIDS. And so we are not completely surprised to see in the popular press pieces like Tim Bugansky's widely syndicated 2007 op-ed piece, "I Miss My Depression."

Sweet melancholy appears as early as John Fletcher's and/or Thomas Middleton's seventeenth-century "Melancholy," which contrasts "sweetest melancholy" to "vain delights." This pattern provides the core characteristic that continues throughout the subsequent centuries. He begins the poem by ordering away these vain delights, which distract him from his conviction that life is incapable of providing enduring satisfaction:

> There 's nought in this life sweet,
> If men were wise to see't
> But only melancholy—
> O sweetest melancholy!

What he is discussing is not (only) some reasoned, philosophical life view, but rather the melancholic construct:

> folded arms and fixèd eyes
> A sigh that piercing mortifies,

> A look that 's fastened to the ground
> A tongue chain'd up without a sound.

In the same era, Robert Burton dwells for many pages of prose on the virtues of melancholy in his ever-lengthening *Anatomy*, having prepared readers for the theme to follow in his upbeat and up-tempo verse "Abstract." Margaret Cavendish elaborates the pattern in her "Discourse on Melancholy," juxtaposing the "chains of passion" with melancholy's "seeming majesty," which pares away distraction to remind us that "only sadness we are apt to keep." In grave matters lies refuge: "What serious is, there constancies will dwell." Yet here again lies more than a detached philosophical stance, as the grave is indeed preferable: "Since death in misery is a release."

The stance is stoic, not in the modern colloquial sense of "put up and shut up" but rather in the classical sense derived from Epictetus, Seneca, Marcus Aurelius, and others who again became widely influential in the Renaissance. In stoic moral thought the well-lived life is one in which the person recognizes his or her proper role and function in the world and lives accordingly. The wise sage is contrasted with the impressionable masses who are constantly distracted from the Good Life by evanescent trivialities that pique their passions and desires. To live free from passions and to accept one's role and function in life is to be truly happy, and truly free.

Not all that takes this stoic stance, though, is melancholy. John Milton's "Il Penseroso" is instructive in its divergence from the melancholic pattern. With its companion, "L'Allegro" (neither included here, for this reason), it provides a compelling inducement to the stoic life. "L'Allegro," ends after over 150 lines in praise of the optimistic, carefree life with a resounding conditional:

> These delights, if thou canst give,
> Mirth with thee, I mean to live.

Thereafter begins "Il Penseroso," with a brusque command: "Hence vain deluding joyes," and it continues thereafter for 173 lines that urge detachment and restraint. It ends with an equally striking (and less conditional) envoi:

> These pleasures Melancholy give,
> And I with thee will choose to live.

Though the term "melancholy" is used throughout, nowhere does the construct appear; instead, here the term designates a philosophical stance.

As might be expected, the sweet melancholy pattern, with various shadings, appears frequently in the Romantics. Some contemporaries, however, dissent. Coleridge's "Dejection" finds little good in the state, and by the end of his "The Suicide's Argument" it is by no means clear which side will win. Clare as well, perhaps having seen too much of the inside of asylums, typically finds the state of little worth; nonetheless, in "To Melancholy" he articulates in a single, final line both its benefit and its cost: "Thy kind face soothes all sorrow save thine own."

In her very distinct style, Dickinson's terse lines and jagged syntax leave the reader to consider, in #435, that "Much Madness is divinest Sense." As in many poems of prior centuries, the poet's "discerning Eye" stands her apart from common knowledge and common sensibility—and this "Majority" is not pleased:

> Assent—and you are sane—
> Demur—you're straightway dangerous—
> And handled with a Chain.

Thus derives the twofold seclusion of the poet: The clarity of vision itself sets the poet apart, and society extrudes and cordons her off.

More recently, but still before the age of modern diagnosis, Edward Thomas's "Melancholy" draws together several of the key themes. Here, and in his more subtly melancholic "Rain," a storm opens the poem. He is driven to solitude by an internal storm: "If I feared the solitude/Far more I feared all company." Alone, he feels the distinct but unnameable emptiness, knowing that all human efforts to assuage the sense will fail. And yet the emptiness itself becomes a manner of fulfillment:

> What I desired I knew not, but whate'er my choice
> Vain it must be, I knew. Yet naught did my despair
> But sweeten the strange sweetness . . .

Hearing a cuckoo and then a waterfall reconnects him with the world around him, though the reconnection leaves him at a slight—yet epochal—remove: He senses

> remote as if in history,
> Rumours of what had touched my friends, my foes, or me.

When we reach the age of modern diagnosis we hear less of the sweetness of melancholy. Perhaps this is in part because modern clinical care and research propose to understand melancholy as a medical disorder and offer alternatives, through treatment, to living with it. Likely more important, though, is the postmodern dissolution of the confidence off earlier ages that, if only one could pierce through the nonsense and vanity of the common life, Truth can be found: In the postmodern world one's truth is another's vanity: there is nothing more to see.

Nonetheless, in the later twentieth century the sweetness still emerges, though obliquely, in a variety of poems. Often it appears only in a subtle, but telling, choice of word or phrase as the poet passes on to apparently different topics, as in Robert Duncan's "Songs of An Other." In this poem the isolated poet, seeking his desired other, is immobilized, "revering strife in a sound of our own" that reaches an inverse crescendo

> toward a conflicting possibility and then
> fury so slowed down it lapses
> into the sweetening melancholy of
>
> a minor key, hovering toward refrain
> it yet refrains from, I come into
> the being of this other me,
>
> exquisitely alone . . .

Theodore Roethke, on the other hand, is much more explicit. It is "In a Dark Time," Roethke tells us, that "the eye begins to see." He asks:

> What's madness but nobility of soul
> At odds with circumstance? The day's on fire!
> I know the purity of pure despair.

Like Duncan, Roethke goes on to perform a pas de deux with an ill-defined shadow, a nebulous other as unidentifiable and unreachable as Edward Thomas's desire is unfulfillable. Yet the endeavor is noble, and melancholy confers on the poet special powers of vision.

Even Plath, so well known as a chronicler of her suffering, recognizes privilege therein. In "Street Song," the jarring image of her flesh that

> Reeks of the butcher's cleaver,
> Its heart and guts hung hooked
> And bloodied

is elevated by messianic allusions:

> thorned hands, feet, head,
> And that great wound
> Squandering red
> From the flayed side,

allowing her, finally, privileged powers of perception that lay bare the secrets of the universe and the non-sense of the common life:

> So, perhaps I, knelled dumb by your absence,
> Alone can hear
> Sun's parched scream,
> Every downfall and crash
> Of gutted star,
> And, more daft than any goose,
> This cracked world's incessant gabble and hiss.

The sweet melancholy pattern is developed in narrative manner in Delmore Schwartz's book-length poem *Genesis*. His protagonist, Hershey Green, is accosted one night by a clutch of spirits. In Book II, unable to sleep and without the comfort of the daytime structures of everyday life, Hershey is overcome with guilt and struck by the senselessness of life. Under the spirits' harpy-like badgering, he cries out to die. The spirits have relentlessly disclosed to him the emptiness of life and—as we have encountered as far back as Fletcher—its "vanity":

> Now we approach the consummation which
> Fulfills and justifies this shameful story,
> Until it must be justified again,
> As human beings, however satisfied,
> By dinner, come for breakfast, until lunch
> Renews the process and prolongs the life,
>   the vanity!

The antidote? To recognize this and to accept the emptiness and look it squarely, dispassionately in the face. In the midst of his hallucination, the poet is driven to the brink of suicide but emerges with new knowledge inaccessible to common folk. To survive he must assume the stoic stance, though without the comfort of the stoic vision of order—more Camus than Epictetus:

> And yet, O New York boy, harsh as this is,
> This is the way to knowledge and to power,
> This is the way to knowledge and to freedom.

Thus the sweetness of melancholy endures in postmodern times—though less frequently, more obliquely, and with no promise of self-evident Truth.

And a handful of other patterns. Other intriguing patterns emerge across poems from very different epochs. Trauma and the response to it are portrayed by tropes as varied as the trauma itself and the epoch. Nonetheless, there recurs a curious pattern reflecting elements of what has clinically been called post-traumatic stress disorder, or PTSD. In poems from the age of modern diagnosis—from Robert L. Barth, Wiley Clements, Lucille Clifton, Richard Hugo, Yusef Komunyakaa, even Anthony Hecht—this may not be surprising. But similar elements appear as well in Siegfried Sassoon's poetry of World War I, an era when the trauma-related response seen in clinics and hospitals was quite different from that seen in the age of modern clinical diagnosis. Some modern features are even evident as early as the beginning of the nineteenth century, for example, in the popular song "Mary Le More."

Additionally, there has also been a long tradition of using madness as a blunt-edged trope or foil for political statements (though such poems are not represented in this volume unless they also have some relevance to the constructs themselves). Madness plays this role in English verse in Jonathan Swift's Mad Mullinix poems, in nineteenth-century popular songs such as "Crazy Paul," and then into the twentieth century in, for example, Hugo's "The Semi-Lunatics of Kilmuir" and certainly in passages from Allen Ginsberg, Carl Solomon, and the other Beats. Les Murray's *Fredy Neptune* provides a book-length poetic account of descent into madness, in Fredy's case hysterical loss of sensation, and ultimate recovery . . . or is it redemption?

Humor also appears across the centuries—in James Carkesse, Robert Fergusson, and the popular songs of the early nineteenth century, and even in Clare's drinking "Song" (though with a bitter aftertaste at the end). In the twentieth century, examples in this anthology come from Dorothy Parker, Theodore Roethke, J. V. Cunningham, Kelly Ann Malone, and others. And what to make of the recurrent, curious sing-songy nursery rhyme–like treatment of madness? Elizabeth Bishop's "Visits to Saint Elizabeths" is perhaps the best known, but there are others: Donald Justice's "Counting the Mad," Anne Sexton's "Ringing the Bells," Stuart Z. Perkoff's sardonic "Junk Nursery Rhymes,"

Edna St. Vincent Millay's "I know a hundred ways to die" (remarkably, actually written for children, since it was included in her *Selected Poems for Young People*), and even back to Thomas Mozeen's "The Bedlamite" in the eighteenth century. And the use of humor in such poems over several centuries raises an interesting question: What *is* so funny about being mad or addicted or suicidal? Sometimes out of the depths comes not a cry but a guffaw.

There are other patterns as well: suicide, mania, heterogeneous views of intoxication and addictions, varied responses to doctors and treatments, and, not least, recovery and its discontents. In addition, issues of gender and madness are evident among the poems of several women represented here, certainly in those of Sexton and Plath, and also as far back as Wroth, Cavendish, and Finch, and as well in Millay's "Menses"—this last sure to stir up debate as heated as any surrounding the *DSM*'s "premenstrual dysphoric disorder."

Thus from our twenty-first-century vantage point a variety of conceptual constructs emerge from written patterns best recognized not in isolated poems but across apparently quite different poems and poets. Identifying these patterns deepens our reading and informs both critical and scientific investigation. Now: Can reading these poems also shed light on Theophrastus's enduring query about the relationship of madness to poetic creativity?

3. Madness and Creativity: Perceiving, Producing

Remarkably robust findings across various scientific studies over the past 150 years demonstrate an association between creativity and some types of mental illness. This is particularly evident for manic-depressive illness, as is well summarized in Kay Redfield Jamison's scholarly yet accessible *Touched with Fire*. The sheer bulk of the research, and parallel discussion in critical circles, indicates that Theophrastus's query engages us still, and merits discussion in the context of these poems.

While a full consideration of the relationship of creativity and these constructs is clearly beyond the scope of a poetry anthology, some traction on the issue is to be gained in the current context. Recall that what we have come to call mental disorders are really best understood as twofold tendencies to *perceive* and to *respond to* the surrounding world in particular ways. The creative process can also be considered a twofold process of *perception* and *response*—of poetic *vision* and poetic *production*. For example, psychiatrist and painter Rollo May in his *Courage to Create* emphasizes the role of the artist as *interpreter* of reality rather than creator de novo of art that somehow springs forth from deep within the artist. Rather, for May perception of the surrounding world is the core of the process. These sentiments echo the earlier considerations of specifically poetic creativity by A. C. Bradley, professor of poetry at Oxford at the turn of the twentieth century: "Poetry . . . , psychologically considered, is not the *expression* of ideas or of a view of life; it is their discovery or creation, or rather both discovery and creation in one" (italics his).[5] We might say, therefore, that perception is the crucial beginning of the creative process, and production follows.

Such a two-step, sequential compartmentalization of tasks is purposely oversimplified. It is meant to be understood conceptually, not chronologically, since the processes of artistic perception and creation are reciprocal, intertwined, and often simultaneous. Yet demarcating these two components conceptually opens the possibility that the constructs we have been considering can have effects on the creative process either by affecting perception, or by affecting production, or both. It necessarily follows that the impact of these constructs needn't be unitary, or even consistent.

The poems that we have discussed illustrate some of the distinct perceptual sets that accompany constructs such as melancholy. For instance, for the melancholic poet the world holds no allure; all is vanity. The poet's remove is radical—even the simple pleasures of the everyday leave the poet cold. The focus turns inward where the sole feeling found therein is the taut ache of emptiness. (One is reminded of Philip Larkin's supposed quip, "What daffodils were to Wordsworth, depression is to me.") The disconnectedness of melancholia stands the poet apart from society and its trivialities. Whether the removal is a product of the poet's stoic resolve or of Isaac Watts's—and modern neuroscientists'—"restless atoms" is the subject of ongoing debate and is, in either case, beside the point: The gap exists.

The poet's withdrawal from the commonsense world—both self-removal and extrusion—produces a vision of the world quite different from that of Dickinson's Majority. But this difference in perception need not necessarily result in (only) a pessimistic, melancholic, dour view of the world. Dissociation from everyday perceptions and preoccupations, from the "vanities" of the commonsense world, permits—stimulates, even—the poet to appreciate a variety of otherwise unnoticed facets of the world.

Of course, melancholy, madness, and the like are not the only paths to such remove. Kurt Vonnegut, in his introduction to the outsider anthology *In the Realms of the Unreal*, suggests that the "mad" writers comprise one among many marginalized groups (including also, for

Vonnegut, women, members of minority populations, and those who have suffered political persecution). The "mad" are certainly among those whom society (not primarily the clinician) culls from its midst. Vonnegut proposes that their experience of being culled from society sets up such individuals for creative perceptions not available to those ensconced in the utilitarian and instrumental demands and strictures of the dominant culture. In another context, William James intuited the human potential for such a two-channel understanding of the world, and indeed considered it to be a core feature of human consciousness: To animals, he suggested, "Sunsets will not suggest heroes' deaths, but only supper-time."[6]

Consider again Edward Thomas's two "rain" poems, "Melancholy" and "Rain." For Thomas, rain is not reduced to its instrumental, production-oriented, Majoritarian functions, such as nourishing crops, filling reservoirs, and making roads slick so that driving gets hazardous. Rather, rain becomes the winnower and the soul cleanser, the vehicle for solitude when it comes, and the harbinger of longing as it clears. For Thomas there is nothing utilitarian, nothing instrumental, about rain—it is instead something at once both personal and transpersonal. Rain is not the territory of meteorologists or engineers or traffic cops.

Nor are such perceptual transformations limited to melancholy. Intoxicants provide another avenue, as Coleridge and various Romantics discovered. More recently, the novelist William Styron in *Darkness Visible* has stated quite explicitly his conviction that his writing declined when his alcoholism remitted. Another example can be found among James Wright's letters, a missive to James Dickey written from Robert Bly's farm, while "drunker than hell . . . here alone in this warm chickenhouse." There he is inspired by "that rare, delicate, magnificent, kind spirit, Gerard de Nerval," and this letter, written, as he says, while under the influence, serves as the nucleus of what would become—at points verbatim—his poem on de Nerval, "In a Warm Chickenhouse."[7]

Mania, too, may have its benefits, and Robert Lowell provides a pivotal example. The plethora of biographies of Lowell and his contemporaries and the recent publication of his copious letters allow us to reconstruct Lowell's personal history in unusual detail (though the more data we have, the more we realize that we still stand at humble remove from Lowell's inner mental life). In editing his letters, Saskia Hamilton takes pains to identify letters written when he was acutely manic. But she also appropriately recognizes the broad range of severity of his episodes. She tells us she will not try to identify his "mildly manic" letters. Her close inspection of his letters and his life had made evident to her the waxing and waning—dimensional—nature of his illness and the impossibility of categorizing discrete periods as "mad" or "sane." When Lowell writes, "I've been furiously writing at poems and spent whole blue and golden Maine days in my bedroom . . . and I have six poems started. They beat the big drum too much," or when Lowell speaks of "the *mystical* experiences and explosions" [italics Lowell's] that "turned out to be pathological and left me . . . inert, gloomy, aimless, vacant, self-locked," is it manic-depression or a creative burst that misses the marks, expands itself, and leaves the poet frustrated and self-doubting? When Lowell speaks of a poem "done mostly when sick" or of another done "while in a long depression," or reports that "the fury of composition had gone" after a three-month "breakdown" that was treated with lithium, we can be somewhat more certain that his illness played a role in his creativity.[8] But we cannot be certain in any categorical sense: mad, manic, hypomanic, hyperthymic, sane—the categories fall short in efforts to understand the *dimensional* role that Lowell's illness played in his creativity. Notwithstanding our inability to pigeonhole his mood excursions, they conferred on him both insight and energy for the creative process. Of this there can be no doubt.

But recall that the creative endeavor is—as are the constructs we have described—processes of both perception *and* response, of both seeing *and* producing. This disaggregated view of the creative process serves to remind us that these two aspects are separable: Poets may write *of* these states, and even write *from* these states, but do they write *in* these states?

The answer is, not surprisingly: it depends. Smart, Clare, James Schuyler, Lowell, and Carruth all wrote while they were institutionalized. Many of those poems have nothing to do with the constructs we have been discussing. (As a side note, in some cases institutionalization may have little to do with madness either, as we are reminded by Fuller Torrey's biography of Ezra Pound and by the legendary peri-institutional exploits of Ginsberg, Solomon, and others among the Beats.) On the other hand, there is clear evidence from the biographies of a variety of poets who were institutionalized or severely ill, as well as from their poems, that they were at times too impaired by mental symptoms to write coherently, let alone brilliantly. (Hear the poets themselves speak of this in, for example, Kenyon's "Having it Out with Melancholy" or Franz Wright's "Thanks Prayer at the Cove.")

To return again to Lowell: His letters make it clear that he despised his illness, and he feared it. He viewed his episodes of mania and depression as aberrations of his character and disruptions in the arc of his poetic work and his life. Though his episodes provided some material for his poems, the most severe excursions of mood were largely destructive to his productivity. Early on in his illness he writes, "I realize that my experiences were like those that might have resulted from a narcotic—terrific lifts, insights, pourings in of new energy, but no work on my part, only more and more self-indulgence, lack of objectivity; and so, into literal madness i.e. I had to be locked up." And in another letter: "In the hospital I spent a mad month or more rewriting *everything* in my three books [italics Lowell's] . . . I felt I had hit the skies, that all cohered. I[t] was mostly waste." Then in a later letter, almost comically: "I went off to the hospital armed with a suit-case of classics: Freud, the complete Aristotle, Dante, etc., and then spent most of my time looking at popular television, even waiting breathlessly for the next Thursday's Dr. Kildare." (Note, though, as an example of the twofold impact of Lowell's manic-depression on his poetic work, that this piece of experience eventually did make its way into his poem "Visitors.")

Finally, suicide: Thomas Lovell Beddoes, John Berryman, Barcroft Boake, Thomas Chatterton, Hart Crane, John Davidson, John Gould Fletcher, Randall Jarrell, Vachel Lindsay, Plath, Sexton, and Sara Teasdale all killed themselves. Clearly madness can inhibit poetic creativity.

To say it briefly: Melancholy, madness, and the like, insofar as they allow the poet to perceive otherwise unnoticed facets of their world, enhance creativity; insofar as they disorganize or paralyze the poet, they impede creativity.

So Theophrastus was right, and now in the twenty-first century we can reconceptualize what he was right about. These states, which some call "madness" and others "mental illness," are not phenomena that open the way to privileged creative realms; neither are they necessarily states that destroy the individual's creative potential. Rather, they are dimensions of human behavior that can support creative perception and productivity, or destroy them—and sometimes both.

Notes

1. Corinne Saunders and Jane Macnaughton, introduction to *Madness and Creativity in Literature and Culture*, ed. Corinne Saunders and Jane Macnaughton (London: Palgrave Macmillan, 2005), p. 5.
2. Geoffrey Hill, *Style and Faith* (New York: Counterpoint Press, 2003), p. 129.
3. Samuel Bownas, *A Description of the Qualifications Necessary to a Gospel Minister* (Philadelphia: Pendle Hill Publications, 1989), p. 5.

4. Plato, *Plato's Phaedrus*, trans. R. Hackforth (New York: Cambridge University Press, 1972), p. 59.

5. A. C. Bradley, *Oxford Lectures on Poetry* (London: Macmillan, 1920), pp. 172–173.

6. William James, *Essays in Psychology* (Harvard University Press, 1983), p. 25.

7. Anne Wright and Saundra Rose Maley, eds., *A Wild Perfection: The Selected Letters of James Wright* (New York: Farrar, Straus & Giroux, 2005), letter to James Dickey, 12/18/60.

8. Saskia Hamilton, ed., *The Letters of Robert Lowell* (New York: Farrar, Straus & Giroux, 2005), letters in order of appearance in the text: to Elizabeth Bishop 9/11/57; to George Santayana, 12/22/49; to Richard Tillinghast, 8/69; ibid.; to Robert Fitzgerald, 8/49; to Elizabeth Bishop, 7/24/59; to Adrienne Rich, 2/25/64.

Selected Bibliography

American Psychiatric Association. *Diagnostic and Statistical Manual of Mental Disorders, Fourth Edition, Text Revision.* Washington, DC: American Psychiatric Press, 2000.

Bownas, Samuel. *A Description of the Qualifications Necessary to a Gospel Minister.* Philadelphia: Pendle Hill Publications, 1989.

Bugansky Tim. "I Miss My Depression." *Boston Globe*, November 20, 2007.

Craddock, Nick, and Michael J. Owen. "The Beginning of the End for the Kraepelinian Dichotomy." *British Journal of Psychiatry* 186 (2005): 364–66.

Engel, George L. "The Need for a New Medical Model: A Challenge for Biomedicine." *Science* 196 (1977): 129–36.

Foucault, Michel. *Madness and Civilization: A History of Insanity in the Age of Reason.* Translated by Richard Howard. New York: Routledge, 1967.

Freud, Sigmund. "Mourning and Melancholia." In *General Psychological Theory: Papers on Metapsychology*, edited by Philip Rieff, 164–179. New York: Touchstone, 1997.

Gilman, Sander L., Helen King, Roy Porter, G. S. Rousseau, and Elaine Showalter. *Hysteria Beyond Freud.* Berkeley: University of California Press, 1993.

Goodwin, Frederick K., and Kay Redfield Jamison. *Manic-Depressive Illness: Bipolar Disorders and Recurrent Depression.* New York: Oxford University Press, 2007.

Gutting, Gary. "Foucault and the History of Madness." In *The Cambridge Companion to Foucault*, 2nd ed., edited by Gary Gutting, 49–73. New York: Cambridge University Press, 2005.

Hamilton, Saskia, ed. *The Letters of Robert Lowell.* New York: Farrar, Straus & Giroux, 2005.

Hill, Geoffrey. *Style and Faith.* New York: Counterpoint Press, 2003.

James, William. *Essays in Psychology.* Cambridge, MA: Harvard University Press, 1983.

Jamison, Kay Redfield. *Exuberance: The Passion for Life.* New York: Alfred A. Knopf, 2004.

———. *Touched with Fire: Manic-Depressive Illness and the Artistic Temperament.* New York: Free Press, 1993.

Kagan, Jerome. "Conceptualizing Psychopathology: The Importance of Developmental Profiles." *Development and Psychopathology* 9 (1997): 321–34.

Kagan, Jerome, and Nancy Snidman. *The Long Shadow of Temperament.* New York: Belknap Press, 2004.

Kendell, Robert E. "What is a Case? Food for Thought for Epidemiologists." *Archives of General Psychiatry* 45 (1988): 374–76.

Kristeva, Julia. *Black Sun: Depression and Melancholia.* Translated by Leon S. Roudiez. New York: Columbia University Press, 1989.

Kupfer, David J., Michael B. First, and Darrel A. Regier, eds. *A Research Agenda for DSM-V.* Washington, DC: American Psychiatric Press, 2005.

May, Rollo. *The Courage to Create.* New York: Norton, 1975.

Moffitt, Terrie E. "The New Look of Behavioral Genetics in Developmental Psychopathology: Gene-Environment Interplay in Antisocial Behaviors." *Psychological Bulletin* 131 (2005): 533–54.

Plato. *Plato's Phaedrus.* Translated by R. Hackforth. New York: Cambridge University Press, 1972.

Porter, Roy. *Madness: A Brief History.* New York: Oxford University Press, 2002.

———. *A Social History of Madness.* London: Weidenfeld & Nicolson, 1987.

Radden, Jennifer, ed. *The Nature of Melancholy from Aristotle to Kristeva.* New York: Oxford University Press, 2000.

Sadler, John Z. *Values and Psychiatric Diagnosis.* New York: Oxford University Press, 2005.

Saudino, Kimberly J. "Behavioral Genetics and Child Temperament." *Journal of Developmental and Behavioral Pediatrics* 26 (2005): 214–23.

Saunders, Corinne, and Jane Macnaughton. Introduction to *Madness and Creativity in Literature and Culture*, edited by Corinne Saunders and Jane Macnaughton. London: Palgrave Macmillan, 2005.

Styron, William. *Darkness Visible.* San Francisco: Chronicle Books, 1992.

Torrey, E. Fuller. *The Roots of Treason: Ezra Pound and the Secret of Saint Elizabeths.* New York: Lucas Publishers, 1999.

Vonnegut, Kurt. Foreword to *In the Realms of the Unreal*, edited by John G. H. Oakes, ix–xi. New York: Four Walls Eight Windows Press, 1991.

World Health Organization. *The ICD-10 Classification of Mental and Behavioural Disorders: Clinical Descriptions and Diagnostic Guidelines.* Geneva, Switzerland: World Health Organization, 1992.

Wright, Anne, and Saundra Rose Maley, eds. *A Wild Perfection: The Selected Letters of James Wright.* New York: Farrar, Straus & Giroux, 2005.

Thomas Hoccleve

(C. 1368–C. 1426)

from "The Complaint of Hoccleve: Hoccleve Remembers His Madness"

Aftir that heruest inned had hise sheues,   *Note: "v" and "u" are used*
And that the broun sesoun of Mihelmesse   *interchangeably. Thus,*
Was come, and gan the trees robbe of her leues *"haruest" is "harvest,"*
That grene had ben and in lusty freisshenesse,   *"sheues" is "sheves"*
And hem into colour of yelownesse   *[sheaves], and, below,*
Had died and doun throwen vndir foote,   *"vnder" is "under"*
That chaunge sanke into myn herte roote.

For freisshly broughte it to my remembraunce
That stablenesse in this worlde is ther noon.
Ther is no thing but chaunge and variaunce.
Howe welthi a man be or wel begoon,
Endure it shal not, he shal it forgoon.
Deeth vndir foote shal him thriste adoun.
That is euery wightes conclucioun,   *wight: fellow*

Wiche for to weyue is in no mannes myght,
Howe riche he be, stronge, lusty, freissh, and gay.
And in the ende of Nouembre vppon a night,
Sighynge sore as I in my bed lay
For this and othir though tis wiche many a day
Byforne I tooke, sleep cam noon in myn ye,
So vexid me the thoughtful maladie.

I sy wel sithin I with siknesse last   *sy: saw; sithin: since*
Was scourgid, cloudy hath bene the fauour
That shoon on me ful bright in times past.
The sunne abated and the dirke shour
Hilded doun right on me and in langour
Me made swymme, so that my spirite
To lyue no lust had ne no delite.

33

The greef aboute myn herte so swal
And bolned euere to and to so sore,   *bolned: surged*
That nedis oute I muste therwithal.
I thoughte I nolde kepe it cloos no more,
Ne lete it in me for to eelde and hore.   *hore: rot*
And for to preue I cam of a womman,
I braste oute on the morwe and thus bigan.   *morwe: morning*

Here endith my prolog and folwith my compleinte

· · ·

And euere sithin, thankid be God oure lord
Of his good and gracious reconsiliacioun,
My wit and I haue bene of suche acord
As we were or the alteracioun
Of it was. But by my sauacioun,
Sith that time haue I be sore sette on fire
And lyued in greet turment and martire.

For though that my wit were hoom come agein,   *hoom: home*
Men wolde it not so vndirstonde or take
With me to dele hadden they disdein.
A rietous persone I was and forsake.
Min oolde frendshipe was al ouershake.
No wight with me list make daliaunce.
The worlde me made a straunge countinaunce,

Wich that myn herte sore gan to tourment.
For ofte whanne I in Westmynstir Halle
And eke in Londoun amonge the prees went,
I sy the chere abaten and apalle
Of hem that weren wonte me for to calle
To companie. Her heed they caste awry
Whanne I hem mette, as they not me sy.

· · ·

'Whanne passinge hete is,' quod thei, 'trustith this,
Assaile him wole agein that maladie.'
And yit, parde, thei token hem amis.
Noon effecte at al took her prophecie.
Manie someris bene past sithen remedie

Of that God of his grace me purueide.
Thankid be God, it shoop not as thei seide.

. . .

And in my chaumbre at home whanne that I was,
Mysilfe aloone I in this wise wrought.
I streite vnto my mirrour and my glas
To loke howe that me of my chere thought,
If any othir were it than it ought.
For fain wolde I if it not had bene right
Amendid it to my kunnynge and might.

Many a saute made I to this mirrour,   *saute: sortie*
Thinking if that I looke in this manere
Amonge folke as I nowe do, noon errour
Of suspecte look may in my face appere.
This countinaunce, I am sure, and this chere
If I it forthe vse is no thing repreuable
To hem that han conceitis resonable.

. . .

I may not lette a man to ymagine
For aboue the mone if that him liste.
Therby the sothe he may not determine,
But by the preef ben thingis knowen and wiste.
Many a doom is wrappid in the myste.
Man bi hise dedis and not be hise lookes
Shal knowen be, as it is writen in bookes.

Bi taaste of fruit men may wel wite and knowe
What that it is. Othir preef is ther noon.
Euery man woote wel that, as that I trowe.
Right so thei that deemen my wit is goon,
As yit this day ther deemeth many oon
I am not wel, may as I by hem goo
Taaste and assay if it be so or noo.

Vppon a look is harde men hem to grounde
What a man is; thereby the sothe is hid.   *sothe: truth*
Whethir hise wittis seek bene or sounde
By countynaunce is it not wist ne kid.
Though a man harde haue oones been bitid,

God shilde it shulde on him contynue alway.   *shilde: shield*
By commvnynge is the beste assay.

I mene to commvne of thingis mene,   *mene: common*
For I am but right lewide douteles   *lewide: lewd*
And ignoraunt. My kunnynge is ful lene.   *lene: lean*
Yit homely resoun knowe I neuerethelees.
Not hope I founden be so resounlees
As men deemen. Marie, Crist forbede!
I can no more. Preue may the dede.

If a man oones falle in drunkenesse,   *oones: once*
Shal he contynue therynne euere mo?
Nay. Though a man do in drinking excesse
So ferforthe that not speke he ne can ne goo
And hise wittis wel ny bene refte him fro
And buried in the cuppe, he aftirward
Cometh to hymsilfe agein. Ellis were it hard.

Rigt so, though that my witte were a pilgrim
And wente fer from home, he cam again.
God me deuoided of the greuous venim
That had enfectid and wildid my brain.
See howe the curteise leche most souerain
Vnto the seke geueth medicine
In nede and hym releueth of his greuous pine.

. . .

'Vexacioun of spirit and turment
Lacke I right noon. I haue of hem plente.
Wondirly bittir is my taast and sent.
Woo be the time of my natiuite!
Vnhappi man, that euere shulde I be!
O deeth, thi strook a salue is of swetnesse
To hem that lyuen in suche wrecchidnesse.

'Gretter plesaunce were it me to die
By manie foolde than for to lyue so.
Sorwes so manie in me multiplie
That my liif is to me a verre foo.
Comforted may I not be of my woo,

Of my distresse see noon ende I can.
No force howe soone I stinte to be a man.'

Thanne spake Resoun: 'What meneth al this fare?
Though welthe be not frendly to thee, yit
Oute of thin herte voide woo and care.'
'By what skile, howe, and by what reed and wit,'
Seide this wooful man, 'mighte I doon it?'
'Wrastle,' quod Resoun, 'agein heuynesse
Of the worlde, troublis, suffringe, and duresse.

'Biholde howe many a man suffrith dissese
As greet as thou, and al away grettere,
And though it hem pinche sharply and sese,
Yit paciently thei it suffre and bere.
Thinke hereon, and the lesse it shal the dere.
Suche suffraunce is of mannes gilte clensinge
And hem enableth to ioie euere lastinge.

'Woo, heuinesse, and tribulacioun
Comen aren to me[n] alle profitable.
Though greuous be mannes temptacioun,
It sleeth man not. To hem that ben suffrable
And to whom Goddis strook is acceptable
Purueied ioie is, for God woundith tho   *ioie: joy*
That he ordeined hath to blis to goo.

'Golde purgid is, thou seest, in the furneis
For the finer and clenner it shal be.
Of thi dissese the weighte and the peis   *peis: heaviness*
Bere lightly, for God to prove the
Scourgid the hath with sharpe aduersite;
Not grucche and seie "Whi susteine I this?"   *grucche: bitterness*
For if thou do, thou the takist amis.

'But thus thou shuldist thinke in thin herte
And seie to thee: "Lorde God, I haue a gilte
So sore I moot for myn offensis smerte
As I am worthi. O lorde, I am spilte
But thou to me thi mercy graunte wilte.

I am ful sure thou maist it not denie.
Lorde, I me repente and I the mercy crie."'

. . .

Farwel my sorwe! I caste it to the cok.
With pacience I hensforthe thinke vnpike
Of suche thoutghtful dissese and woo the lok
And lete hem out that han me made to sike.
Hereafter oure lorde God may if him like
Make al myn oolde affeccioun resorte,
And in hope of that wole I me comforte.

. . .

∽

from "Anxious Thought"

MUSING upon the restless bisynesse
    The which this troubly world hath ay on hande,
That other thing than fruit of bitternesse
    Ne yeeldeth not, as I can understande,
    At Chestres Inne, right faste by the Strande,
      As I lay in my bed upon a night,
      Thought me bereft of sleep the force and might.

. . .

So long a night ne felt I never none
    As was that same, to my juggement.
Whoso that thoughty is, he is wo-begone;
    The thoughtful wight is vessel of torment:
    Ther is no greef to him equipollent:
      He graveth deepest of sicknesses alle—
      Ful wo is him that in such cas is falle.

What wight that inly pensif is, I trowe,   *inly: within; trowe: believe*
    His moste desire is to be solitarie;
That this is sooth in my persone I knowe,

For ever whil that fretting adversarie
Mine hertë madë to him tributàrie
   In souking of the freshest of my blood,
   To sorwe soole me thought it did me good

      . . .

When to the thoughtful wight is told a tale,
   He heereth it as though he thenne were;
His hevy thoughtes so him plukke and hale   *hale: heave*
   Hider and thider, and him greve and dere,   *dere: hurt*
   That his eres availe him not a pere: *pere: pear*
      He understandeth nothing what men saye,
      So been his wittes gone fro him awaye.

The smert of thought I by experience
   Knowe also wel as doth any man living:
His frosty swote and firy-hot fervence   *swote: sweat*
   And troubly dremes, drempt al in waking,
   My mazed hed sleepless han of cunning
      And wit despoiled, and so me bejaped
      That after deth ful often have I gaped.

Charles d'Orleans

(1394–1465)

I am Forsaken

Care away, away, away,
   Murninge away!
I am forsake, another is take;
   No more murne ich may.   *Ich: I*

I am sory for her sake,
   Ich may wel ete and drinke;
When ich slepe ich may not wake,
   So muche on her ich thinke.

I am brought in such a bale
   And brought in such a pine,
When ich rise up of my bed
   Me liste wel to dine.

I am brought in suche a pine,
   Y-brought in such a bale,
When ich have right good wine
   Me Liste drinke non ale.

Farewell this World

Farewell, this world! I take my leve for evere;
I am arested to apere at Goddes face.
O myghtyfull God, thou knowest that I had levere
Than all this world to have oone houre space
To make asythe for all my grete trespace.

40

My hert, alas, is brokyne for that sorowe—
Som be this day that shall not be tomorow!

This lyfe, I see, is but a cheyre feyre;
All thyngis passene and so most I algate.
Today I sat full ryall in a cheyere,
Tyll sotell Deth knokyd at my gate,
And onavysed he seyd to me, 'Chek-mate!'
Lo, how sotell he maketh a devors!
And, wormys to fede, he hath here leyd my cors.

Speke softe, ye folk, for I am leyd aslepe!
I have my dreme—in trust is moche treson.
Fram Dethes hold feyne wold I make a lepe,
But my wysdom is turnyd into feble resoun:
I see this worldis joye lastith but a season—
Wold to God I had remembyrd me beforne!
I sey no more, but be ware of ane horne!

This febyll world, so fals and so unstable,
Promoteth his lovers for a lytell while,
But at the last he yeveth hem a bable
When his peynted trowth is torned into gile.
Experyence cawsith me the trowth to compile,
Thynkyng this, to late, alas, that I began,
For foly and hope disseyveth many a man.

Farewell, my frendis! the tide abidith no man:
I moste departe hens, and so shall ye.
But in this passage, the beste song that I can
Is *Requiem eternam*—I pray God grant it me!
Whan I have endid all myn adversite,
Graunte me in Paradise to have a mancyon,
That shede his blode for my redempcion.

41

William Dunbar

(1460–1520)

In Winter

Into thir dirk and drublie dayis	*drublie: turbid*
Quhone sabill all the hevin arrayis	*Quhone: when; sabill: black*
With mystie vapouris, cluddis, and skyis,	
Nature all curage me denyis	
Off sangis, ballattis, and of playis.	*sangis: songs; ballattis: ballads*

Quhone that the nycht dois lenthin houris
With wind, with haill, and havy schouris,
    My dulé spreit dois lurk for schoir;
    My hairt for languor dois forloir
For laik of Symmer with his flouris.

I walk, I turne, sleip may I nocht;	
I vexit am with havie thocht,	
This warld all ovir I cast about,	
And ay the mair I am in dout	*mair: more*
The mair that I remeid have socht.	

I am assayit on everie syde:
Dispair sayis, 'Ay in tyme provyde
    And get sum thing quharion to leif,
    Or with grit trouble and mischeif
Thow sall into this court abyd.'

Than Patience sayis, 'Be not agast:
Hald Hoip and Treuthe within the fast,
    And lat Fortoun wirk furthe hir rage,
    Quhome that no rasoun may assuage
Quhill that hir glas be run and past.'

And Prudence in my eir sayis ay,
'Quhy wald thow hald that will away?

Or craif that thow may have mo space,
Thow tending to ane uther place
A journay going everie day?'

And than sayis Age, 'My friend, cum neir,
And be not strange, I the requeir:
Cum, brodir, by the hand me tak,
Remember thow hes compt to mak
Off all thi tyme thow spendit heir.'

Syne Deid castis upe his yettis wyd,   *wyd: wood*
Saying, 'Thir oppin sall the abyd;   *abyd: abide*
Albeid that thow wer neuer sa stout,
Undir this lyntall sall thow lowt:
Thair is nane uther way besyde.'

For feir of this all day I drowp;
No gold in kist, nor wyne in cowp,
No ladeis bewtie, nor luiffis blys,
May lat me to remember this,
How glaid that ever I dyne or sowp.   *sowp: sup*

Yit, quhone the nycht begynnis to schort,
It dois my spreit sumpairt confort,
Off thocht oppressit with the schowris.   *schowris: showers*
Cum, lustie Symmer, with thi flowris,
That I may leif in sum disport.

Alexander Barclay

(1475–1552)

from "The Ship of Fools—Of Glotons and Dronkardes"

. . .

Some sowe-dronke, swaloynge mete without mesure,
Some mawdelayne dronke, mournynge lowdly and hye,
Some beynge dronke no lenger can endure
Without they gyve them to bawdy rybawdry;
Some swereth armys, nayles, herte and body,
Terynge our Lord worse than the Jowes hym arayed;
Some nought can speke, but harkenyth what is sayd.

Some spende all that they have and more at wast
With 'revell and revell, dasshe fyll the cup Joohn!'
Some their thryft lesyth with dyce at one cast;
Some slepe as slogardes tyll their thryft be gone,
Some shewe theyr owne counsell for kepe can they none,
Some are ape-dronke, full of lawghter and of toyes,
Some mery dronke, syngynge with wynches and boyes.

Some spue, some stacker, some utterly ar lame,
Lyeng on the grounde without power to ryse;
Some bost them of bawdry, ferynge of no shame;
Some dumme, and some speketh wordes at thryse;
Some charge theyr bely with wyne in such wyse
That theyr legges skant can bere up the body—
Here is a sort to drowne a hole navy!

Anonymous

(published 1500)

A Song of Ale

Back and side go bare, go bare,
   Both hand and foot go cold,
But belly, God send thee good ale enough
   Whether it be new or old!

But if that I may have truly
   Good ale my belly full,
I shall look like one, by sweet Saint John,
   Were shorn against the wool.
Though I go bare, take you no care,
   I am nothing a-cold,
I stuff my skin so full within
   Of jolly good ale and old.

I cannot eat but little meat,
   My stomach is not good;
But sure I think that I could drink
   With him that weareth an hood.
Drink is my life; although my wife
   Some time do chide and scold,
Yet spare I not to ply the pot
   Of jolly good ale and old.

I love no roast but a brown toast,
   Or a crab in the fire;
A little bread shall do me stead;
   Much bread I never desire.
Nor frost, nor snow, nor wind I trow,
   Can hurt me if it would,
I am so wrapped within and lapped
   With jolly good ale and old.

I care right nought, I take no thought
　　For clothes to keep me warm;
Have I good drink, I surely think
　　Nothing can do me harm:
For truly than I fear no man,
　　Be he never so bold,
When I am armed and thoroughly warmed
　　With jolly good ale and old.

But now and than I curse and ban,
　　They make their ale so small;
God give them care and evil to fare!
　　They stry the malt and all.
Such peevish pew, I tell you true,
　　Not for a crown of gold,
There cometh one sip within my lip,
　　Whether it be new or old.

Good ale and strong maketh me among
　　Full jocund and full light,
That oft I sleep and take no keep
　　From morning until night.
Then start I up and flee to the cup;
　　The right way on I hold;
My thirst to staunch, I fill my paunch
　　With jolly good ale and old.

And Kit my wife, that as her life
　　Loveth well good ale to seek,
Full oft drinketh she, that ye may see
　　The tears run down her cheek.
Then doth she troll to me the bowl,
　　As a good malt-worm should,
And say 'Sweet-heart, I have take my part
　　Of jolly good ale and old.'

They that do drink till they nod and wink,
　　Even as good fellows should do,
They shall not miss to have the bliss,
　　That good ale hath brought them to.

And all poor souls that scour black bowls,
    And them hath lustily trolled,
God save the lives of them and their wives,
    Whether they be young or old!

Petition to Have Her Leave to Die

When will the fountain of my tears be dry?
    When will my sighs be spent?
When will desire agree to let me die?
    When will thy heart relent?
It is not for my life I plead,
Since death the way to rest doth lead;
        But stay for thy consent,
        Lest thou be discontent.

For if myself without thy leave I kill,
    My ghost will never rest;
So hath it sworn to work thine only will,
    And holds that ever best;
For since it only lives by thee,
Good reason thou the ruler be.
        Then give me leave to die,
        And show thy power thereby.

Fulke Greville

(1554–1628)

from "Despair"

Who grace for zenith had,
  From which no shadows grow,
Who hath seen joy of all his hopes
  And end of all his woe;

Whose love beloved hath been
  The crown of his desire,
Who hath seen sorrow's glories burnt
  In sweet affection's fire;

If from this heavenly state,
  Which souls with souls unites,
He be fallen down into the dark
Despaired war of sprights;

Let him lament with me,
  For none doth glory know,
That hath not been above himself,
  And thence fallen down to woe.

But if there be one hope
  Left in his languished heart,
If fear of worse, if wish of ease,
  If horror may depart;

He plays with his complaints,
  He is no mate for me,
Whose love is lost, whose hopes are fled,
  Whose fears for ever be.

. . .

My winter is within,
  Which withereth my joy,
My knowledge seat of civil war,
  Where friends and foes destroy;

And my desires are wheels,
  Whereon my heart is borne,
With endless turning of themselves,
  Still living to be torn.

My thoughts are eagles' food,
  Ordained to be a prey
To worth; and being still consumed,
  Yet never to decay.

My memory, where once
  My heart laid up the store
Of help, of joy, of spirit's wealth,
  To multiply them more,

Is now become the tomb
  Wherein all these lie slain,
My help, my joy, my spirit's wealth,
  All sacrificed to pain.

In paradise I once
  Did live and taste the tree,
Which shadowed was from all the world,
  In joy to shadow me.

The tree hath lost his fruit,
  Or I have lost my seat;
My soul both black with shadow is
  And over-burnt with heat.

Truth here for triumph serves
  To show her power is great,
Whom no desert can overcome,
  Nor no distress entreat.

Time past lays up my joy,
    And time to come my grief;
She ever must be my desire
    And never my relief.

Wrong her lieutenant is;
    My wounded thoughts are they,
Who have no power to keep the field,
    Nor will to run away.

O rueful constancy,
    And where is change so base,
As it may be compared with thee
    In scorn and in disgrace?

· · ·

Since then this is my state,
    And nothing worse than this,
Behold the map of death-like life,
    Exiled from lovely bliss.

Alone among the world,
    Strange with my friends to be,
Showing my fall to them that scorn,
    See not or will not see;

My heart a wilderness,
    My studies only fear,
And, as in shadows of curst death,
    A prospect of despair;

My exercise must be
    My horrors to repeat,
My peace, joy, end, and sacrifice
    Her dead love to entreat;

My food the time that was,
    The time to come my fast,
For drink the barren thirst I feel
    Of glories that are past;

Sighs and salt tears my bath,
   Reason my looking-glass,
To show me he most wretched is,
   That once most happy was;

Forlorn desires my clock,
   To tell me every day,
That time hath stolen love, life, and all
   But my distress away;

For music heavy signs,
   My walk an inward woe,
Which like a shadow ever shall
   Before my body go.

And I myself am he
   That doth with none compare,
Except in woes and lack of worth,
   Whose states most wretched are.

Let no man ask my name,
   Nor what else I should be;
For *Griev-Ill*, pain, forlorn estate,
   Do best decipher me.

Thomas Lodge

(1557–1625)

Melancholy

The earth, late choked with showers,
   Is now arrayed in green;
Her bosom springs with flowers,
   The air dissolves her teen:
The heavens laugh at her glory,
Yet bide I sad and sorry.

The woods are decked with leaves,
   And trees are clothed gay;
And Flora, crowned with sheaves,
   With oaken boughs doth play:
Where I am clad in black,
The token of my wrack.

The birds upon the trees
   Do sing with pleasant voices,
And chant in their degrees
   Their loves and lucky choices:
When I, whilst they are singing,
With sighs mine arms am wringing.

The thrushes seek the shade,
   And I my fatal grave;
Their flight to heaven is made,
   My walk on earth I have:
They free, I thrall; they jolly,
I sad and pensive wholly.

William Shakespeare

(1564–1616)

Sonnet 129

Th' expense of spirit in a waste of shame
Is lust in action; and, till action, lust
Is perjured, murderous, bloody full of blame,
Savage, extreme, rude, cruel, not to trust,
Enjoyed no sooner but despisèd straight,
Past reason hunted, and no sooner had
Past reason hated as a swallowed bait
On purpose laid to make the taker mad.
Mad in pursuit, and in possession so;
Had, having, and in quest to have, extreme;
A bliss in proof, and proved, a very woe,
Before a joy proposed; behind, a dream.
All this the world well knows, yet none knows well
To shun the heaven that leads men to this hell.

Sir Henry Wotton

(1568–1639)

Upon the Death of Sir Albert Morton's Wife

He first deceased; she for a little tried
   To live without him, liked it not, and died.

A Hymn to My God in a Night of My Late Sickness

O thou great power, in whom I move,
For whom I live, to whom I die,
Behold me through thy beams of love,
Whilst on this couch of tears I lie;
   And cleanse my sordid soul within
   By thy Christ's blood, the bath of sin.

No hallowed oils, no grains I need,
No rags of saints, no purging fire,
One rosy drop from David's seed
Was worlds of seas, to quench thine ire.
   O precious ransom! which once paid,
   That *Consummatum est* was said:

And said by him that said no more,
But sealed it with his sacred breath.
Thou then, that has dispunged my score,
And dying, wast the death of death,
   Be to me now, on thee I call,
   My life, my strength, my joy, my all.

Sir John Davies

(1569–1618)

Affliction

If aught can teach us aught, Affliction's looks,
    Making us look into ourselves so near,
Teach us to know ourselves beyond all books,
    Or all the learned schools that ever were.

This mistress lately plucked me by the ear,
    And many a golden lesson hath me taught;
Hath made my senses quick, and reason clear,
    Reformed my will, and rectified my thought.

So do the winds and thunders cleanse the air;
    So working seas settle and purge the wine;
So lopped and pruned trees do flourish fair;
    So doth the fire the drossy gold refine.

Neither Minerva nor the learned Muse,
    Nor rules of art, nor precepts of the wise,
Could in my brain those beams of skill infuse,
    As but the glance of this dame's angry eyes.

She within lists my ranging mind hath brought,
    That now beyond myself I list not go;
Myself am centre of my circling thought,
    Only myself I study, learn, and know.

I know my body's of so frail a kind
    As force without, fevers within, can kill;
I know that heavenly nature of my mind,
    But 'tis corrupted both in wit and will;

I know my soul hath power to know all things,
    Yet is she blind and ignorant in all;

I know I am one of nature's little kings,
   Yet to the least and vilest things am thrall.

I know my life's a pain and but a span,
   I know my sense is mocked with everything;
And to conclude, I know myself a man,
   Which is a proud, and yet a wretched thing.

Robert Burton

(1577–1640)

The Author's Abstract of Melancholy

When I go musing all alone
Thinking of divers things fore-known.
When I build castles in the air,
Void of sorrow and void of fear,
Pleasing myself with phantasms sweet,
Methinks the time runs very fleet.
 All my joys to this are folly,
  Naught so sweet as melancholy.
When I lie waking all alone,
Recounting what I have ill done,
My thoughts on me then tyrannise,
Fear and sorrow me surprise,
Whether I tarry still or go,
Methinks the time moves very slow.
 All my griefs to this are jolly,
  Naught so mad as melancholy.
When to myself I act and smile,
With pleasing thoughts the time beguile,
By a brook side or wood so green,
Unheard, unsought for, or unseen,
A thousand pleasures do me bless,
And crown my soul with happiness.
 All my joys besides are folly,
  None so sweet as melancholy.
When I lie, sit, or walk alone,
I sigh, I grieve, making great moan,
In a dark grove, or irksome den,
With discontents and Furies then,
A thousand miseries at once
Mine heavy heart and soul ensconce,
 All my griefs to this are jolly,
  None so sour as melancholy.

Methinks I hear, methinks I see,
Sweet music, wondrous melody,
Towns, palaces, and cities fine;
Here now, then there; the world is mine,
Rare beauties, gallant ladies shine,
Whate'er is lovely or divine.
    All other joys to this are folly,
    None so sweet as melancholy.
Methinks I hear, methinks I see
Ghosts, goblins, fiends; my phantasy
Presents a thousand ugly shapes,
Headless bears, black men, and apes,
Doleful outcries, and fearful sights,
My sad and dismal soul affrights.
    All my griefs to this are jolly,
    None so damn'd as melancholy.
Methinks I court, methinks I kiss,
Methinks I now embrace my mistress.
O blessed days, O sweet content,
In Paradise my time is spent.
Such thoughts may still my fancy move,
So may I ever be in love.
    All my joys to this are folly,
    Naught so sweet as melancholy.
When I recount love's many frights,
My sighs and tears, my waking nights,
My jealous fits; O mine hard fate
I now repent, but 'tis too late.
No torment is so bad as love,
So bitter to my soul can prove.
    All my griefs to this are jolly,
    Naught so harsh as melancholy.
Friends and companions get you gone,
'Tis my desire to be alone;
Ne'er well but when my thoughts and I
Do domineer in privacy.
No Gem, no treasure like to this,
'Tis my delight, my crown, my bliss.
    All my joys to this are folly,
    Naught so sweet as melancholy.
'Tis my sole plague to be alone,

I am a beast, a monster grown,
I will no light nor company,
I find it now my misery.
The scene is turn'd, my joys are gone,
Fear, discontent, and sorrows come.
    All my griefs to this are jolly,
    Naught so fierce as melancholy.
I'll not change life with any king,
I ravisht am: can the world bring
More joy, than still to laugh and smile,
In pleasant toys time to beguile?
Do not, O do not trouble me,
So sweet content I feel and see.
    All my joys to this are folly,
    None so divine as melancholy.
I'll change my state with any wretch,
Thou canst from gaol or dunghill fetch;
My pain's past cure, another hell,
I may not in this torment dwell!
Now desperate I hate my life,
Lend me a halter or a knife;
    All my griefs to this are jolly,
    Naught so damn'd as melancholy.

John Fletcher and/or Thomas Middleton

(1579–1625; 1580–1627)

Melancholy

Hence, all you vain delights,
  As short as are the nights
  Wherein you spend your folly!
There's naught in this life sweet,
If men were wise to see't,
  But only melancholy—
  O sweetest melancholy!
Welcome, folded arms and fixèd eyes,
A sigh that piercing mortifies,
A look that 's fasten'd to the ground,
A tongue chain'd up without a sound!

Fountain-heads and pathless groves,
Places which pale passion loves!
Moonlight walks, when all the fowls
Are warmly housed, save bats and owls!
  A midnight bell, a parting groan—
  These are the sounds we feed upon:
Then stretch our bones in a still gloomy valley,
Nothing 's so dainty sweet as lovely melancholy.

Lady Mary Wroth

(1586–c. 1652)

Sonnet XIX from *The Countess of Montgomery's Urania*

COME, darkest night, becoming sorrow best;
  Light, leave thy light, fit for a lightsome soul;
  Darkness doth truly suit with me oppressed,
  Whom absence' power doth from mirth control:
The very trees with hanging heads condole
  Sweet summer's parting, and of leaves distressed
  In dying colours make a griefful roll,
  So much, alas, to sorrow are they pressed.
Thus of dead leaves her farewell carpet's made:
  Their fall, their branches, all their mournings prove,
  With leafless, naked bodies, whose hues vade
  From hopeful green, to wither in their love:
If trees and leaves for absence mourners be,
No marvel that I grieve, who like want see.

Sonnet VI from *Pamphilia to Amphilanthus*

My paine still smother'd in my grieved brest,
  Seekes for some ease, yet cannot passage finde,
  To be discharged of this unwelcome guest,
  When most I strive, more fast his burthens binde.
Like to a Ship on Goodwins cast by winde,
  The more shee strive, more deepe in Sand is prest,
  Till she be lost: so am I in this kind
  Sunck, and devour'd, and swallow'd by unrest.

Lost, shipwrackt, spoyld, debar'd of smallest hope,
  Nothing of pleasure left, save thoughts have scope,
  Which wander may; goe then my thoughts and cry:
Hope's perish'd, Love tempest-beaten, Joy lost,
  Killing Despaire hath all these blessings crost;
  Yet Faith still cries, Love will not falsifie.

Robert Herrick

(1591–1674)

The Mad Maid's Song

GOOD-MORROW to the day so fair,
   Good-morning, sir, to you;
Good-morrow to mine own torn hair
   Bedabbled with the dew.

Good-morning to this primrose too,
   Good-morrow to each maid
That will with flowers the tomb bestrew
   Wherein my love is laid.

Ah! woe is me, woe, woe is me!
   Alack and well-a-day!
For pity, sir, find out that bee
   Which bore my love away.

I'll seek him in your bonnet brave,
   I'll seek him in your eyes;
Nay, now I think they've made his grave
   I' th' bed of strawberries.

I'll seek him there; I know ere this
   The cold, cold earth doth shake him;
But I will go, or send a kiss
   By you, sir, to awake him.

Pray hurt him not; though he be dead,
   He knows well who do love him,
And who with green turfs rear his head,
   And who do rudely move him.

He's soft and tender (pray take heed);
   With bands of cowslips bind him,
And bring him home—but 'tis decreed
   That I shall never find him!

George Herbert

(1593–1633)

Affliction (I)

WHEN first Thou didst entice to Thee my heart,
    I thought the service brave:
So many joys I writ down for my part,
    Besides what I might have
Out of my stock of naturall delights,
Augmented with Thy gracious benefits.

I lookèd on Thy furniture so fine,
    And made it fine to me;
Thy glorious household stuff did me entwine,
    And 'tice me unto Thee.
Such stars I counted mine: both heaven and earth
Paid me my wages in a world of mirth.

What pleasures could I want, whose King I served,
    Where joys my fellows were?
Thus argued into hopes, my thoughts reserved
    No place for grief or fear;
Therefore my sudden soul caught at the place,
And made her youth and fierceness seek Thy face:

At first thou gavest me milk and sweetnesses;
    I had my wish and way:
My days were strewed with flowers and happiness:
    There was no month but May.
But with my years sorrow did twist and grow,
And made a party unawares for woe.

My flesh began unto my soul in pain,
    Sicknesses clave my bones,
Consuming agues dwell in every vein,
    And tune my breath to groans,

Sorrow was all my soul; I scarce believed,
Till grief did tell me roundly, that I lived.

When I got health, Thou took'st away my life—
    And more; for my friends die:
My mirth and edge was lost: a blunted knife
    Was of more use than I.
Thus, thin and lean, without a fence or friend,
I was blown through with every storm and wind.

Whereas my birth and spirit rather took
    The way that takes the town,
Thou didst betray me to a lingering book,
    And wrap me in a gown.
I was entangled in the world of strife,
Before I had the power to change my life.

Yet, for I threatened oft the siege to raise,
    Not simpering all mine age,
Thou often didst with academic praise
    Melt and dissolve my rage.
I took thy sweetened pill, till I came near;
I could nor go away, nor persevere.

Yet, lest perchance I should too happy be
    In my unhappiness,
Turning my purge to food, Thou throwest me
    Into more sicknesses.
Thus doth Thy power cross-bias me, not making
Thine own gift good, yet me from my ways taking.

Now I am here, what thou wilt do with me
    None of my books will show:
I read, and sigh, and wish I were a tree—
    For sure, then, I should grow
To fruit or shade; at least, some bird would trust
Her household to me, and I should be just.

Yet, though Thou troublest me, I must be meek;
    In weakness must be stout:
Well, I will change the service, and go seek
    Some other master out.

Ah, my dear God! though I am clean forgot,
Let me not love Thee, if I love Thee not.

Affliction (IV)

Broken in pieces all asunder,
Lord, hunt me not,
A thing forgot,
Once a poor creature, now a wonder,
A wonder tortur'd in the space
Betwixt this world and that of grace.

My thoughts are all a case of knives,
Wounding my heart
With scatter'd smart,
As wat'ring pots give flowers their lives.
Nothing their fury can control,
While they do wound and prick my soul.

All my attendants are at strife,
Quitting their place
Unto my face:
Nothing performs the task of life:
The elements are let loose to fight,
And while I live, try out their right.

Oh help, my God! let not their plot
Kill them and me,
And also thee,
Who art my life: dissolve the knot,
As the sun scatters by his light
All the rebellions of the night.

Then shall those powers, which work for grief,
Enter thy pay,

And day by day
Labour thy praise, and my relief;
With care and courage building me,
Till I reach heav'n, and much more, thee.

 ❧

The Collar

 I struck the board, and cried, "No more
I will abroad.
What! shall I ever sigh and pine?
My lines and life are free; free as the road,
Loose as the wind, as large as store.
Shall I be still in suit?
Have I no harvest but a thorn
To let me blood, and not restore
What I have lost with cordial fruit?
Sure there was wine
Before my sighs did dry it; there was corn
Before my tears did drown it.
Is the year only lost to me?
Have I no bays to crown it?
No flowers, no garlands gay? all blasted?
All wasted?
Not so, my heart; but there is fruit,
And thou hast hands.
Recover all thy sigh-blown age
On double pleasures; leave thy cold dispute
Of what is fit and not; forsake thy cage,
Thy rope of sands,
Which petty thoughts have made, and made to thee
Good cable, to enforce and draw,
And be thy law,
While thou didst wink and wouldst not see.
Away! take heed;
I will abroad.
Call in thy death's-head there; tie up thy fears;

He that forbears
To suit and serve his need
Deserves his load."
But as I rav'd, and grew more fierce and wild
At every word,
Me thoughts I heard one calling, "Child";
And I replied, "My Lord."

John Milton

(1608–1674)

from "Samson Agonistes"

. . .

Samson:
All otherwise to me my thoughts portend,
That these dark orbs no more shall treat with light,
Nor th' other light of life continue long,
But yield to double darkness nigh at hand:
So much I feel my genial spirits droop,
My hopes all flat, nature within me seems
In all her functions weary of her self;
My race of glory run, and race of shame,
And I shall shortly be with them that rest.
    Manoa [Samson's father]:
Believe not these suggestions which proceed
From anguish of the mind and humours black,
That mingle with thy fancy. I however
Must not omit a Fathers timely care
To prosecute the means of thy deliverance
By ransom or how else: mean while be calm,
And healing words from these thy friends admit.
    Samson:
O that torment should not be confin'd
To the bodies wounds and sores
With maladies innumerable
In heart, head, brest, and reins;
But must secret passage find
To th' inmost mind,
There exercise all his fierce accidents,
And on her purest spirits prey,
As on entrails, joints, and limbs,
With answerable pains, but more intense,
Though void of corporal sense.
My griefs not only pain me

As a lingring disease,
But finding no redress, ferment and rage,
Nor less then wounds immedicable
Ranckle, and fester, and gangrene,
To black mortification.
Thoughts my Tormenters arm'd with deadly stings
Mangle my apprehensive tenderest parts,
Exasperate, exulcerate, and raise
Dire inflammation which no cooling herb
Or medcinal liquor can asswage,
Nor breath of Vernal Air from snowy *Alp*.
Sleep hath forsook and giv'n me o're
To deaths benumming Opium as my only cure.
Thence faintings, swounings of despair,
And sense of Heav'ns desertion.

. . .

⌒

"Methought I saw my late espousèd Saint"

Methought I saw my late espousèd Saint
   Brought to me like *Alcestis* from the grave,
   Whom *Joves* great Son to her glad Husband gave,
   Rescu'd from death by force though pale and faint.
Mine as whom washt from spot of child-bed taint,
   Purification in the old Law did save,
   And such, as yet once more I trust to have
   Full sight of her in Heaven without restraint,
Came vested all in white, pure as her mind:
   Her face was vail'd, yet to my fancied sight,
   Love, sweetness, goodness in her person shin'd
So clear, as in no face with more delight.
   But O as to embrace me she inclin'd,
   I wak'd, she fled, and day brought back my night.

70

Anne Bradstreet

(1612–1672)

Upon Some Distemper of the Body

In anguish of my heart replete with woes,
And wasting pains, which best my body knows,
In tossing slumbers on my wakeful bed,
Bedrenched with tears that flowed from mournful head,
Till nature had exhausted all her store,
Then eyes lay dry, disabled to weep more;
And looking up unto his throne on high,
Who sendeth help to those in misery;
He chased away those clouds and let me see
My anchor cast i' th' vale with safety.
He eased my soul of woe, my flesh of pain,
and brought me to the shore from troubled main.

Margaret Cavendish, Duchess of Newcastle

(1624–1674)

A Discourse on Melancholy

A sad and solemn verse doth please the mind,
With chains of passions doth the spirits bind.
As pencilled pictures drawn presents the night,
Whose darker shadows give the eye delight,
Melancholy aspects invite the eye,
And always have a seeming majesty.
By its converting qualities there grows
A perfect likeness, when itself it shows.
Then let the world in mourning sit and weep,
Since only sadness we are apt to keep.
In light and toyish things we seek for change;
The mind grows weary, and about doth range.
What serious is, there constancies will dwell;
Which shows that sadness mirth doth far excel.
Why should men grieve when they do think of death,
Since they no settlement can have in mirth?
The grave, though sad, in quiet still they keep:
Without disturbing dreams they lie asleep,
No rambling thoughts to vex their restless brains,
Nor labour hard, to scorch and dry their veins.
No care to search for that they cannot find,
Which is an appetite to every mind.
Then wish, good man, to die in quiet peace,
Since death in misery is a release.

Thomas Traherne

(1636–1674)

Solitude

How desolate!
Ah! how forlorn, how sadly did I stand
   When in the field my woful State
      I felt! Not all the Land,
         Not all the Skies,
   Tho Heven shin'd before mine Eys,
Could Comfort yield in any Field to me,
Nor could my Mind Contentment find or see.

   Remov'd from Town,
From People, Churches, Feasts, and Holidays,
   The Sword of State, the Mayor's Gown,
      And all the Neighb'ring Boys;
         As if no Kings
   On Earth there were, or living Things,
The silent Skies salute mine Eys, the Seas
My Soul surround; no Rest I found, or Eas.

   My roving Mind
Search'd evry Corner of the spacious Earth,
   From Sky to Sky, if it could find,
      (But found not) any Mirth:
         Not all the Coasts,
   Nor all the great and glorious Hosts,
In Hev'n or Earth, did any Mirth afford;
No welcom Good or needed Food, my Board.

   I do believ,
The Ev'ning being shady and obscure,
   The very Silence did me griev,
      And Sorrow more procure:
         A secret Want
   Did make me think my Fortune scant.

73

I was so blind, I could not find my Health,
No Joy mine Ey could there espy, nor Wealth.

    Nor could I ghess
What kind of thing I long'd for: But that I
  Did somwhat lack of Blessedness,
    Beside the Earth and Sky,
      I plainly found;
  It griev'd me much, I felt a Wound
Perplex me sore; yet what my Store should be
I did not know, nothing would shew to me.

    Ye sullen Things!
Ye dumb, ye silent Creatures, and unkind!
  How can I call you Pleasant Springs
    Unless ye eas my Mind!
      Will ye not speak
  What 'tis I want, nor Silence break?
O pity me, and let me see som Joy;
Som Kindness shew to me, altho a Boy.

    They silent stood;
Nor Earth, nor Woods, nor Hills, nor Brooks, nor Skies,
  Would tell me where the hidden Good,
    Which I did long for, lies:
      The shady Trees,
  The Ev'ning dark, the humming Bees,
The chirping Birds, mute Springs and Fords, conspire,
While they deny to answer my Desire.

    Bells ringing I
Far off did hear, som Country Church they spake;
  The Noise re-ecchoing throu the Sky
    My Melancholy brake;
      When't reacht mine Ear
  Som Tidings thence I hop'd to hear:
But not a Bell me News could tell, or shew
My longing Mind, where Joys to find, or know.

    I griev'd the more,
'Caus I therby somwhat encorag'd was

That I from thence should learn my Store;
    For Churches are a place
      That nearer stand
   Than any part of all the Land
To Hev'n; from whence som little Sense I might
To help my Mind receiv, and find som Light.

     They louder sound
Than men do talk, somthing they should disclose;
   The empty Sound did therfore wound
     Becaus not shew Repose.
       did revive
   To think that Men were there alive;
But had my Soul, call'd by the Toll, gon in,
I might have found, to eas my Wound, a Thing.

     A little Eas
Perhaps, but that might more molest my Mind;
   One flatt'ring Drop would more diseas
     My Soul with Thirst, and grind
      My Heart with grief:
   For People can yield no Relief
In publick sort when in that Court they shine,
Except they mov my Soul with Lov divine.

     Th' External Rite,
Altho the face be wondrous sweet and fair,
   Can satiate my Appetit
     No more than empty Air
      Yield solid Food.
   Must I the best and highest Good
Seek to possess; or Blessedness in vain
(Tho 'tis alive in som place) strive to gain?

     O! what would I
Diseased, wanting, melancholy, giv
   To find *that* tru Felicity,
     The place where Bliss doth liv?
      Those Regions fair
   Which are not lodg'd in Sea nor Air,
Nor Woods, nor Fields, nor Arbour yields, nor Springs,
Nor Hev'ns shew to us below, nor Kings.

I might hav gon
Into the City, Market, Tavern, Street,
    Yet only chang'd my Station,
        And strove in vain to meet
            That Eas of Mind
    Which all alone I long'd to find:
A common Inn doth no such thing betray,
Nor doth it walk in Peeple's Talk, or Play.

        O Eden fair!
Where shall I seek the Soul of Holy Joy
    Since I to find it here despair;
        Nor in the shining Day,
            Nor in the Shade,
    Nor in the Field, nor in a Trade
I can it see? Felicity! O where
Shall I thee find to eas my Mind! O where!

James Carkesse

(published 1679)

On the Doctors' Telling Him that till He Left off Making Verses He Was Not Fit to be Discharged

Desiring his imprisoned Muse to enlarge,
The poet, Mad-quack moved, for his discharge.
He angry answered, 'Parson, 'tis too soon:
As yet I have not cured you of lampoon;
For know, New Bedlam chiefly for the infected
With this new sort of madness was erected:
Bucks both and Rochester, unless they mend,
Hither the king designs forthwith to send.
Shepherd and Dryden too must on 'em wait;
For he's resolved at once to rid the state
Of this poetic, wanton, madlike tribe,
Whose rampant Muse does court and city gibe.
Thus Bedlam may be cured perchance, if it hits,
After despair of physic, by the wits.'
The answer pleased; yet I have cause to fear
The doctor flattered, as 'tis usual here.
But if my brethren come, I've learned this lesson:
In such good company, Bedlam is no prison.

Anonymous

(published 1658)

On Melancholy

Stand off, physician! Let me frolic
With my humour melancholic.
   'Tis pleasure–it is pain likewise;
   'Tis hell, and yet a paradise.
'Tis white and black—'tis all upon
Checkered imagination.
   'Tis an odd-conceited theme;
   'Tis nature's rambling, idle dream;
Her cheating optic glass, which lies,
Falsely abstracts, and multiplies.

The man of Rhodes, whose stature was
Nine hundred camels' load of brass,
   This mighty Phoebus can't compare
   With the melancholy I bear,
In hands, feet, nose—fancy makes him
Bigger by far in every limb.

Another wasteful humour straight
Brings him down to a half-ounce weight,
   Then, like some bird (a pretty folly!)
   Flies aloft, winged with melancholy!
He's air, or some thin exhalation
Next degree to annihilation.

'Tis thraldom, freedom, 'tis express
Good company, and loneliness;
   It laughs and cries all in one breath;
   'Tis wealth or want, 'tis life or death.
A Bedlam trance, 'tis what you will,
'Tis as you'd have it, well or ill.

A fickle contradicting mood,
Arising from distempered blood

Stand off, physician! 'Tis, I'm sure,
As a disease, so its own cure.

Anne Finch, Countess of Winchilsea

(1661–1720)

The Spleen: A Pindaric Poem

What art thou, spleen, which ev'ry thing dost ape
Thou Proteus to abus'd Mankind,
Who never yet thy real Cause cou'd find,
Or fix thee to remain in one continued Shape.
Still varying thy perplexing Form,
Now a Dead Sea thou'lt represent,
A Calm of stupid Discontent,
Then, dashing on the Rocks wilt rage into a Storm.
Trembling sometimes thou dost appear,
Dissolv'd into a Panick Fear;
On Sleep intruding dost thy Shadows spread,
Thy gloomy Terrours round the silent Bed,
And croud with boading Dreams the Melancholy Head:
Or, when the Midnight Hour is told,
And drooping Lids thou still dost waking hold,
Thy fond Delusions cheat the Eyes,
Before them antick Spectres dance,
Unusual Fires their pointed Heads advance,
And airy Phantoms rise.
Such was the monstrous Vision seen,
When Brutus (now beneath his Cares opprest,
And all Rome's Fortunes rolling in his Breast,
Before Philippi's latest Field,
Before his Fate did to Octavius lead)
Was vanquish'd by the Spleen.

Falsly, the Mortal Part we blame
Of our deprest, and pond'rous Frame,
Which, till the First degrading Sin
Let Thee, its dull Attendant, in,
Still with the Other did comply,
Nor clogg'd the Active Soul, dispos'd to fly,

And range the Mansions of it's native Sky.
Nor, whilst in his own Heaven he dwelt,
Whilst Man his Paradice possest,
His fertile Garden in the fragrant East,
And all united Odours smelt,
No armed Sweets, until thy Reign,
Cou'd shock the Sense, or in the Face
A flusht, unhandsom Colour place.
Now the Jonquille o'ercomes the feeble Brain;
We faint beneath the Aromatick Pain,
Till some offensive Scent thy Pow'rs appease,
And Pleasure we resign for short, and nauseous Ease.

In ev'ry One thou dost possess,
New are thy Motions, and thy Dress:
Now in some Grove a list'ning Friend
Thy false Suggestions must attend,
Thy whisper'd Griefs, thy fancy'd Sorrows hear,
Breath'd in a Sigh, and witness'd by a Tear;
Whilst in the light, and vulgar Croud,
Thy Slaves, more clamorous and loud,
By Laughters unprovok'd, thy Influence too confess.
In the Imperious Wife thou Vapours art,
Which from o'erheated Passions rise
In Clouds to the attractive Brain,
Until descending thence again,
Thro' the o'er-cast, and show'ring Eyes,
Upon her Husband's soften'd Heart,
He the disputed Point must yield,
Something resign of the contested Field;
Til Lordly Man, born to Imperial Sway,
Compounds for Peace, to make that Right away,
And Woman, arm'd with Spleen, do's servilely Obey.

The Fool, to imitate the Wits,
Complains of thy pretended Fits,
And Dulness, born with him, wou'd lay
Upon thy accidental Sway;
Because, sometimes, thou dost presume
Into the ablest Heads to come:
That, often, Men of Thoughts refin'd,

Impatient of unequal Sence,
Such slow Returns, where they so much dispense,
Retiring from the Croud, are to thy Shades inclin'd.
O'er me, alas! thou dost too much prevail:
I feel thy Force, whilst I against thee rail;
I feel my Verse decay, and my crampt Numbers fail.
Thro' thy black Jaundice I all Objects see,
As Dark, and Terrible as Thee,
My Lines decry'd, and my Employment thought
An useless Folly, or presumptuous Fault:
Whilst in the Muses Paths I stray,
Whilst in their Groves, and by their secret Springs
My Hand delights to trace unusual Things,
And deviates from the known, and common way;
Nor will in fading Silks compose
Faintly th' inimitable Rose,
Fill up an ill-drawn Bird, or paint on Glass
The Sov'reign's blurr'd and undistinguish'd Face,
The threatning Angel, and the speaking Ass.

Patron thou art to ev'ry gross Abuse,
The sullen Husband's feign'd Excuse,
When the ill Humour with his Wife he spends,
And bears recruited Wit, and Spirits to his Friends.
The Son of Bacchus pleads thy Pow'r,
As to the Glass he still repairs,
Pretends but to remove thy Cares,
Snatch from thy Shades one gay, and smiling Hour,
And drown thy Kingdom in a purple Show'r.
When the Coquette, whom ev'ry Fool admires,
Wou'd in Variety be Fair,
And, changing hastily the Scene
From Light, Impertinent, and Vain,
Assumes a soft, a melancholy Air,
And of her Eyes rebates the wand'ring Fires,
The careless Posture, and the Head reclin'd,
The thoughtful, and composed Face,
Proclaiming the withdrawn, the absent Mind,
Allows the Fop more liberty to gaze,
Who gently for the tender Cause inquires;
The Cause, indeed, is a Defect in Sense,
Yet is the Spleen alleg'd, and still the dull Pretence.

But these are thy fantastic Harms,
The Tricks of thy pernicious Stage,
Which do the weaker Sort engage;
Worse are the dire Effects of thy more pow'rful Charms.
By Thee Religion, all we know,
That shou'd enlighten here below,
Is veil'd in Darkness, and perplext
With anxious Doubts, with endless Scruples vext,
And some Restraint imply'd from each perverted Text.

Whilst Touch not, Taste not, what is freely giv'n,
Is but thy niggard Voice, disgracing bounteous Heav'n.
From Speech restrain'd, by thy Deceits abus'd,
To Desarts banish'd, or in Cells reclus'd,
Mistaken Vot'ries to the Pow'rs Divine,
Whilst they a purer Sacrifice design,
Do but the Spleen obey, and worship at thy Shrine.
In vain to chase thee ev'ry Art we try,
In vain all Remedies apply,
In vain the Indian Leaf infuse,
Or the parch'd Eastern Berry bruise;
Some pass, in vain, those Bounds, and nobler Liquors use.
Now Harmony, in vain, we bring,
Inspire the Flute, and touch the String.
From Harmony no help is had;
Musick but soothes thee, if too sweetly sad,
And if too light, but turns thee gayly Mad.

Tho' the Physicians greatest Gains,
Altho' his growing Wealth he sees
Daily increas'd by Ladies Fees,
Yet dost thou baffle all his studious Pains.
Not skilful Lower thy Source cou'd find,
Or thro' the well-dissected Body trace
The secret, the mysterious ways,
By which thou dost surprize, and prey upon the Mind.
Tho' in the Search, too deep for Humane Thought,
With unsuccessful Toil he wrought,
'Til thinking Thee to've catch'd, Himself by thee was caught,
Retain'd thy Pris'ner, thy acknowleg'd Slave,
And sunk beneath thy Chain to a lamented Grave.

Edward Ward

(1667–1731)

The Extravagant Drunkard's Wish

Had I my Wish I would distend my Guts
   As wide as from the North to Southern Skies,
And have, at once, as many Mouths and Throats,
   As old Briarius Arms, or Argos Eyes.
The raging Sea's unpallatable Brine,
   That drowns so many Thousands in a Year,
I'd turn into an Ocean of good Wine,
   And for my Cup would chuse the Hemisphere:
Would then perform the Wager Xanthus laid,
   In spight of all the Rivers flowing Streams,
Swill, till I piss'd a Deluge, then to Bed,
   And please my thirsty Soul with Small-Beer Dreams.
Thus Drink and Sleep, and waking Swill again,
   Till I had drunk the Sea-Gods Cellars dry,
Then rob the Niggard Neptune and his Train
   Of Tritons, of that Wealth they now enjoy.
Kiss the whole Nerides, and make the Jades
   Sing all their charming Songs to please my Ear,
And whether Flesh or Fish, Thornbacks or Maids,
   I'd make the Gypsies kind thro' Love or Fear.
And when thus Wicked and thus Wealthy grown
   For nothing good, I'd turn Rebellious Whig,
Pull e'ery Monarch headlong from his Throne,
   And with the Prince of Darkness make a League,
That he and I, and all the Whigs beside,
   Might rend down Churches, Crowns in pieces tare,
Exert our Malice, gratify our Pride,
   And settle Satan's Kingdom e'erywhere.

Isaac Watts

(1674–1748)

The Hurry of the Spirits, in a Fever and Nervous Disorders

My frame of nature is a ruffled sea,
And my disease the tempest. Nature feels
A strange commotion to her inmost centre;
The throne of reason shakes. 'Be still, my thoughts;
Peace and be still.' In vain my reason gives
The peaceful word, my spirit strives in vain
To calm the tumult and command my thoughts.
This flesh, this circling blood, these brutal powers,
Made to obey, turn rebels to the mind,
Nor hear its laws. The engine rules the man.
Unhappy change! When nature's meaner springs,
Fir'd to impetuous ferments, break all order;
When little restless atoms rise and reign
Tyrants in sov'reign uproar, and impose
Ideas on the mind; confus'd ideas
Of non-existents and impossibles,
Who can describe them? Fragments of old dreams,
Borrow'd from midnight, torn from fairy fields
And fairy skies, and regions of the dead,
Abrupt, ill-sorted! O 'tis all confusion!
If I but close my eyes, strange images
In thousand forms and thousand colours rise,
Stars, rainbows, moons, green dragons, bears and ghosts,
An endless medley rush upon the stage,
And dance and riot wild in reason's court
Above control. I'm in a raging storm,
Where seas and skies are blended, while my soul
Like some light worthless chip of floating cork
Is tost from wave to wave: Now overwhelm'd
With breaking floods, I drown, and seem to lose
All being: Now high-mounted on the ridge

Of a tall foaming surge, I'm all at once
Caught up into the storm, and ride the wind,
The whistling wind; unmanageable steed,
And feeble rider! Hurried many a league
Over the rising hills of roaring brine,
Thro' airy wilds unknown, with dreadful speed
And infinite surprise; till some few minutes
Have spent the blast, and then perhaps I drop
Near to the peaceful coast; some friendly billow
Lodges me on the beach, and I find rest:
Short rest I find; for the next rolling wave
Snatches me back again; then ebbing far
Sets me adrift, and I am borne off to sea,
Helpless, amidst the bluster of the winds,
Beyond the ken of shore.

Ah, when will these tumultuous scenes be gone?
When shall this weary spirit, tost with tempests,
Harass'd and broken, reach the port of rest,
And hold it firm? When shall this wayward flesh
With all th'irregular springs of vital movement
Ungovernable, return to sacred order,
And pay their duties to the ruling mind?

Edward Young

(1683–1765)

from "Night Thoughts on Life, Death, and Immortality: Night I"

Tired Nature's sweet restorer, balmy Sleep!
He, like the world, his ready visit pays
Where Fortune smiles; the wretched he forsakes;
Swift on his downy pinion flies from woe,
And lights on lids unsullied with a tear.

From short (as usual) and disturb'd repose
I wake: how happy they who wake no more!
Yet that were vain, if dreams infest the grave.
I wake, emerging from a sea of dreams
Tumultuous; where my wreck'd desponding thought,
From wave to wave of fancied misery,
At random drove, her helm of reason lost:
Though now restored, 'tis only change of pain,
(A bitter change!) severer for severe.
The Day too short for my distress; and Night,
E'en in the zenith of her dark domain,
Is sunshine to the colour of my fate.

Night, sable goddess! from her ebon throne,
In rayless majesty, now stretches forth
Her leaden sceptre o'er a slumbering world.
Silence, how dead! and darkness, how profound!
Nor eye, nor listening ear, an object finds;
Creation sleeps. 'Tis as the general pulse
Of life stood still, and Nature made a pause;
An awful pause! prophetic of her end.
And let her prophecy be soon fulfill'd:
Fate! drop the curtain; I can lose no more.

. . .

This is the desert, this the solitude:
How populous, how vital is the grave!
This is creation's melancholy vault,
The vale funereal, the sad cypress-gloom;
The land of apparitions, empty shades!
All, all on earth is shadow, all beyond
Is substance; the reverse is Folly's creed:
How solid all, where change shall be no more!
This is the bud of being, the dim dawn,
The twilight of our day, the vestibule:
Life's theatre as yet is shut, and Death,
Strong Death, alone can heave the massy bar,
This gross impediment of clay remove,
And make us embryos of existence free.
From real life but little more remote
Is he, not yet a candidate for light,
The future embryo, slumb'ring in his sire.
Embryos we must be till we burst the shell,
Yon ambient azure shell, and spring to life,
The life of gods (O transport!) and of man.

William Harrison

(1685–1713)

In Praise of Laudanum

I feel, O Laudanum, thy power divine,
And fall with pleasure at thy slumb'ring shrine:
Lulled by thy charms I 'scape each anxious thought,
And everything but Mira is forgot.

Mary Barber

(1685–1755)

On seeing an Officer's Widow distracted, who had been driven to Despair by a long and fruitless Solicitation for the Arrears of her Pension

O wretch! Hath madness cured thy dire despair?
Yes—All thy sorrows now are light as air:
No more you mourn your once loved husband's fate,
Who bravely perished for a thankless state.
For rolling years thy piety prevailed;
At length, quite sunk—thy hope, thy patience failed.
Distracted now you tread on life's last stage,
Nor feel the weight of poverty and age:
How blest in this, compared with those whose lot
Dooms them to miseries, by you forgot!
   Now, wild as winds, you from your offspring fly,
Or fright them from you with distracted eye;
Rove through the streets; or sing, devoid of care,
With tattered garments and dishevelled hair;
By hooting boys to higher frenzy fired,
At length you sink, by cruel treatment tired,
Sink into sleep, an emblem of the dead,
A stone thy pillow, the cold earth thy bed.
   O tell it not; let none the story hear,
Lest Britain's martial sons should learn to fear:
And when they next the hostile wall attack,
Feel the heart fail, the lifted arm grow slack;
And pausing cry—'Though death we scorn to dread,
Our orphan offspring, must they pine for bread?
See their loved mothers into prisons thrown,
And, unrelieved, in iron bondage groan?'
   Britain, for this impending ruin dread;
Their woes call loud for vengeance on thy head:
Nor wonder, if disasters wait your fleets;
Nor wonder at complainings in your streets.
Be timely wise; arrest th' uplifted hand,
Ere pestilence or famine sweep the land.

Anonymous

(published 1692)

Loving Mad Tom

I'll bark against the Dog-star,
And crow away the morning;
   I'll chase the moon
   Till it be noon,
And I'll make her leave her horning.
But I will find Bonny Maud, Merry Mad Maud,
   And seek whate'er betides her;
     Yet I will love
     Beneath or above
   That dirty Earth that hides her.

I'll crack the poles asunder,
   Strange things I will devise on.
I'll beat my brain against Charles's Wain,
   And I'll grasp the round horizon.
But I will find Bonny Maud, Merry Mad Maud,
   And seek whate'er betides her;
     Yet I will love
     Beneath or above
   That dirty Earth that hides her.

I'll search the caves of slumber,
   And please her in a night dream;
I'll tumble her into Lawrence's fen,
   And hang myself in a sunbeam;
But I will find Bonny Maud, Merry Mad Maud,
   And seek whate'er betides her;
     Yet I will love
     Beneath or above
   That dirty Earth that hides her.

I'll sail upon a millstone,
   And make the sea-gods wonder;

I'll plunge in the deep, till I wake asleep,
   And I'll tear the rocks in sunder.
But I will find Bonny Maud, Merry Mad Maud,
   And seek whate'er betides her;
     Yet I will love
     Beneath or above
   That dirty Earth that hides her.

Matthew Green

(1696–1737)

from **"The Spleen. An Epistle to Mr. C—— J——"**

. . .

First know, my friend, I do not mean
To write a treatise on the Spleen;
Nor to prescribe when nerves convulse;
Nor mend th'alarum watch, you pulse.
If I am right, your question lay,
What course I take to drive away
The day-mare Spleen, by whose false pleas
Men prove mere suicides in ease;
And how I do myself demean
In stormy world to live serene.

When by its magick lantern Spleen
With frightful figures spreads life's scene,
And threat'ning prospects urg'd my fears,
A stranger to the luck of heirs;
Reason, some quiet to restore,
Shew'd part was substance, shadow more;
With Spleen's dead weight tho' heavy grown,
In life's rough tide I sunk not down,
But swam, till Fortune threw a rope,
Buoyant on bladders fill'd with hope.

I always choose the plainest food
To mend viscidity of blood.
Hail! water-gruel, healing power,
Of easy access to the poor;
Thy help love's confessors implore,
And doctors secretly adore;
To thee I fly, by thee dilute—
Thro' veins my blood doth quicker shoot,
And by swift current throws off clean
Prolifick particles of Spleen.

I never sick by drinking grow,
Nor keep myself a cup too low,
And seldom Cloe's lodgings haunt,
Thrifty of spirits, which I want.

Hunting I reckon very good
To brace the nerves, and stir the blood;
But after no field-honours itch,
Atchiev'd by leaping hedge and ditch.
While Spleen lies soft relax'd in bed,
Or o'er coal fires inclines the head,
Hygeia's sons with hound and horn,
And jovial cry awake the morn.
These see her from the dusky plight,
Smear'd by th'embraces of the night,
With roral wash redeem her face,
And prove herself of Titan's race,
And, mounting in loose robes the skies,
Shed light and fragrance as she flies.
Then horse and hound fierce joy display,
Exulting at the Hark-away,
And in pursuit o'er tainted ground
From lungs robust field-notes resound.
Then, as St. George the dragon slew,
Spleen pierc'd, trod down, and dying view;
While all their spirits are on wing,
And woods, and hills, and vallies ring.

To cure the mind's wrong biass, Spleen;
Some recommend the bowling-green;
Some, hilly walks; all, exercise;
Fling but a stone, the giant dies;
Laugh and be well. Monkeys have been
Extreme good doctors for the Spleen;
And kitten, if the humour hit,
Has harlequin'd away the fit.

Since mirth is good in this behalf,
At some partic'lars let us laugh.

. . .

In rainy days keep double guard,
Or Spleen will surely be too hard;
Which, like those fish by sailors met,
Fly highest, while their wings are wet.
In such dull weather, so unfit
To enterprize a work of wit,
When clouds one yard of azure sky,
That's fit for simile, deny,
I dress my face with studious looks,
And shorten tedious hours with books.
But if dull fogs invade the head,
That mem'ry minds not what is read,
I sit in window dry as ark,
And on the drowning world remark:
Or to some coffee-house I stray
For news, the manna of a day,
And from the hipp'd discourses gather,
That politicks go by the weather:
Then seek good-humour'd tavern chums,
And play at cards, but for small sums;
Or with the merry fellows quaff,
And laugh aloud with them that laugh;
Or drink a joco-serious cup
With souls who've took their freedom up,
And let my mind, beguil'd by talk,
In Epicurus' garden walk,
Who thought it heav'n to be serene,
Pain hell; and purgatory spleen.

Sometimes I dress, with women sit,
And chat away the gloomy fit;
Quit the stiff garb of serious sense,
And wear a gay impertinence,
Nor think, nor speak with any pains,
But lay on fancy's neck the reins;
Talk of unusual swell of waist
In maid of honour loosely lac'd,
And beauty borr'wing Spanish red,
And loving pair with sep'rate bed,
And jewels pawn'd for loss of game,
And then redeem'd by loss of fame;

Of Kitty (aunt left in the lurch
By grave pretence to go to church)
Perceiv'd in hack with lover fine,
Like Will and Mary on the coin:
And thus in modish manner we,
In aid of sugar, sweeten tea.

. . .

William Collins

(1721–1759)

Ode to Fear

Strophe:

Thou, to whom the world unknown
With all its shadowy shapes is shown;
Who see'st appalled the unreal scene,
While Fancy lifts the veil between:
   Ah Fear! Ah frantic Fear!
   I see, I see thee near.
I know thy hurried step, thy haggard eye!
Like thee I start, like thee disordered fly.
For lo, what monsters in thy train appear!
Danger, whose limbs of giant mould
What mortal eye can fixed behold?
Who stalks his round, an hideous form,
Howling amidst the midnight storm,
Or throws him on the ridgy steep
Of some loose hanging rock to sleep;
And with him thousand phantoms joined,
Who prompt to deeds accursed the mind;
And those, the fiends who, near allied,
O'er nature's wounds and wrecks preside;
Whilst Vengeance in the lurid air
Lifts her red arm, exposed and bare,
On whom that ravening brood of fate,
Who lap the blood of sorrow, wait;
Who, Fear, this ghastly train can see,
And look not madly wild like thee?

Epode:

In earliest Greece to thee with partial choice
   The grief-full Muse addressed her infant tongue;

The maids and matrons on her awful voice,
   Silent and pale, in wild amazement hung.

Yet he, the bard who first invoked thy name,
   Disdained in Marathon its power to feel:
For not alone he nursed the poet's flame,
   But reached from Virtue's hand the patriot's steel.

But who is he whom later garlands grace,
   Who left awhile o'er Hybla's dews to rove,
With trembling eyes thy dreary steps to trace,
   Where thou and Furies shared the baleful grove?

Wrapped in thy cloudy veil the incestuous queen
   Sighed the sad call her son and husband heard,
When once alone it broke the silent scene,
   And he, the wretch of Thebes, no more appeared.

O Fear, I know thee by my throbbing heart,
   Thy withering power inspired each mournful line,
Though gentle Pity claim her mingled part,
   Yet all the thunders of the scene are thine!

Antistrophe:

Thou who such weary lengths hast passed,
Where wilt thou rest, mad nymph, at last?
Say, wilt thou shroud in haunted cell,
Where gloomy Rape and Murder dwell?
Or in some hollowed seat,
'Gainst which the big waves beat,
Hear drowning seamen's cries in tempests brought!
Dark power, with shuddering meek submitted thought
Be mine to read the visions old,
Which thy awakening bards have told:
And, lest thou meet my blasted view,
Hold each strange tale devoutly true;
Ne'er be I found, by thee o'erawed,
In that thrice-hallowed eve abroad,
When ghosts, as cottage-maids believe,
Their pebbled beds permitted leave,

And goblins haunt, from fire or fen
Or mine or flood, the walks of men!
O thou whose spirit most possessed
The sacred seat of Shakespeare's breast!
By all that from thy prophet broke,
In thy divine emotions spoke,
Hither again thy fury deal,
Teach me but once like him to feel:
His cypress wreath my meed decree,
And I, O Fear, will dwell with thee!

Thomas Mozeen

(published 1768)

The Bedlamite

'Tis not on the face displayed,
  What I suffer, cruel maid!
A burning poison lurks unseen:
  O ease me; ease my sad chagrin!
See through yon fiery lake, yon flaming flood,
Fierce dragons come to drink my blood.
      Why, Jove, dost thou thus set them on?
       O what have I done,
       My dear, dear, dazzling sun,
        That no wind from the sea
        Blows tidings to me,
       Whilst the tyrant frowns on my throne?

Shall we to the meadows go,
  Where the butter-flowers blow,
And the dainty daisies grow?
        I say No, no, no, no, no, no.
For lend me a while your ear;
     How can I be merry,
     Whilst you guzzle sherry,
And I must sip small beer?——

     Give me the reward,
     Give me the reward;
And fill the goblet high:
I now the traitor spy;——
      Tread soft and fair,
      All light as air,
      'Tis my belief,
      Yon plantain leaf
Conceals him from your eye.

'Tis a Spaniard on my life!——
Tawny face——bloody knife!——
But let the bells merrily ring;
  We have store of great guns,
  And fine Chelsea buns,
  And the burgundy runs;
And we love and we honour the King.

Nay, be not so harsh with your smiles;
  Your frowns are more pleasant to me.
Hark! hearken to puss on the tiles!——
  She's just such a lady as thee.

Ah Fanny! Why dost thou so sadly complain?
Thou canst not sure envy my temperate brain.
    Off, off the course,
    That damned trotting horse:
    I'll hold six to four
    You hear on't no more;
For Prussia has beat them again.——

  Of reason I held a lease,
But long, very long 't has been out:
  O landlord, renew, if you please!
Help, counsellor——bring it about.
  What!——Nothing without your fees?——
Ah, tickle me not for a trout.——

    How now, saucy Jack;
    Why appear'st thou in black?——
A packet to me, say'st, directed;
    Ha! ha! ha! ha!
    Bow, enemies, bow!
    Or I'll harass you now:
'Tis the comet so long we've expected.——

Nay, soothe me not; for well I know,
To cure my tortured heart of woe
  Is not to mortal given:
She only can my sense restore
Who robbed me of it once before;
  An angel, no in heaven.

Christopher Smart

(1722–1771)

Hymn to the Supreme Being, on Recovery from a Dangerous Fit of Illness

To DOCTOR *JAMES*

I

When
Israel's ruler on the royal bed
  In anguish and in perturbation lay,
The down reliev'd not his anointed head,
  And rest gave place to horror and dismay.
Fast flow'd the tears, high heav'd each gasping sigh
When God's own prophet thunder'd—MONARCH, THOU
  MUST DIE.

II

And must I go, th'illustrious mourner cry'd,
  I who have serv'd thee still in faith and truth,
Whose snow-white conscience no foul crime has died
  From youth to manhood, infancy to youth,
Like *David*, who have still rever'd thy word
The sovereign of myself and servant of the Lord!

III

The judge Almighty heard his suppliant's moan,
  Repeal'd his sentence, and his health restor'd;
The beams of mercy on his temples shone,
  Shot from that heaven to which his sighs had soar'd;
The sun retreated at his maker's nod
And miracles confirm the genuine work of God.

IV

But, O immortals! What had I to plead
  When death stood o'er me with his threat'ning lance,

When reason left me in the time of need,
    And sense was lost in terror or in trance,
My sinking soul was with my blood inflam'd,
And the celestial image sunk, defac'd and maim'd,

V
I sent back memory, in heedful guise,
    To search the records of preceding years;
Home, like the raven to the ark, she flies,
    Croaking bad tidings to my trembling ears.
O sun, again that thy retreat was made,
And threw my follies back into the friendly shade!

VI
But who are they, that bid affliction cease!—
    Redemption and forgiveness, heavenly sounds!
Behold the dove that brings the branch of peace,
    Behold the balm that heals the gaping wounds—
Vengeance divine's by penitence supprest
She struggles with the angel, conquers, and is blest.

VII
Yet hold, presumption, nor too fondly climb,
    And thou too hold, O horrible despair!
In man humility's alone sublime,
    Who diffidently hopes he's *Christ*'s own care—
O all-sufficient Lamb! in death's dread hour
Thy merits who shall slight, or who can doubt thy power?

VIII
But soul-rejoicing health again returns,
    The blood meanders gentle in each vein,
The lamp of life renew'd with vigour burns,
    And exil'd reason takes her seat again—
Brisk leaps the heart, the mind's at large once more,
To love, to praise, to bless, to wonder and adore.

IX
The virtuous partner of my nuptial bands,
    Appear'd a widow to my frantic sight;

My little prattlers lifting up their hands,
  Beckon me back to them, to life, and light;
I come, ye spotless sweets! I come again,
Nor have your tears been shed, nor have ye knelt in vain.

X

All glory to th'eternal, to th'immense,
  All glory to th'omniscient and good,
Whose power's uncircumscrib'd, whose love's intense;
  But yet whose justice ne'er could be withstood.
Except thro' him—thro' him, who stands alone,
Of worth, of weight allow'd for all Mankind t'atone!

XI

He rais'd the lame, the lepers he made whole,
  He fix'd the palsied nerves of weak decay,
He drove out Satan from the tortur'd soul,
  And to the blind gave or restor'd the day,—
Nay more,—far more unequal'd pangs sustain'd,
Till his lost fallen flock his taintless blood regain'd.

XII

My feeble feet refus'd my body's weight,
  Nor wou'd my eyes admit the glorious light,
My nerves convuls'd shook fearful of their fate,
  My mind lay open to the powers of night.
He pitying did a second birth bestow
A birth of joy—not like the first of tears and woe.

XIII

Ye strengthen'd feet, forth to his altar move;
  Quicken, ye new-strung nerves, th'enraptur'd lyre;
Ye heav'n-directed eyes, o'erflow with love;
  Glow, glow, my soul, with pure seraphic sire;
Deeds, thoughts, and words no more his mandates break,
But to his endless glory work, conceive, and speak.

XIV

O! penitence, to virtue near allied,
  Thou can'st new joys e'en to the blest impart;
The list'ning angels lay their harps aside
  To hear the musick of thy contrite heart;

And heav'n itself wears a more radiant face,
When charity presents thee to the throne of grace.

XV

Chief of metallic forms is regal gold;
　　Of elements, the limpid fount that flows;
Give me 'mongst gems the brilliant to behold;
　　O'er *Flora*'s flock imperial is the rose:
Above all birds the sov'reign eagle soars;
And monarch of the field the lordly lion roars.

XVI

What can with great *Leviathan* compare,
　　Who takes his pastime in the mighty main?
What, like the *Sun*, shines thro' the realms of air,
　　And gilds and glorifies th'ethereal plain—
Yet what are these to man, who bears the sway;
For all was made for him—to serve and to obey.

XVII

Thus in high heaven charity is great,
　　Faith, hope, devotion hold a lower place;
On her the cherubs and the seraphs wait,
　　Her, every virtue courts, and every grace;
See! on the right, close by th'Almighty's throne,
In him she shines confest, who came to make her known.

XVIII

Deep-rooted in my heart then let her grow,
　　That for the past the future may atone;
That I may act what thou hast giv'n to know,
　　That I may live for thee and thee alone,
And justify those sweetest words from heav'n,
"That he shall love thee most to whom thou'st most forgiven. . . ."

from "Jubilate Agno," Fragment B

Let Elizur rejoice with the Partridge, who is a prisoner of state and
is proud of his keepers.
*For I am not without authority in my jeopardy, which I derive
inevitably from the glory of the name of the Lord.*

Let Shedeur rejoice with Pyrausta, who dwelleth in a medium of fire,
which God hath adapted for him.
*For I bless God whose name is Jealous—and there is a zeal to deliver us
from everlasting burnings.*

Let Shelumiel rejoice with Olor, who is of a goodly savour, and the
very look of him harmonizes the mind.
*For my existimation is good even amongst the slanderers and my
memory shall arise for a sweet savour unto the Lord.*

Let Jael rejoice with the Plover, who whistles for his live, and foils the
marksmen and their guns.
*For I bless the PRINCE of PEACE and pray that all the guns may be
nail'd up, save such as are for the rejoicing days.*

Let Raguel rejoice with the Cock of Portugal—God send good Angels
to the allies of England!
*For I have abstained from the blood of the grape and that even at the
Lord's table.*

Let Hobab rejoice with Necydalus, who is the Greek of a Grub.
*For I have glorified God in GREEK and LATIN, the consecrated
languages spoken by the Lord on earth.*

Let Zurishaddai with the Polish Cock rejoice—The Lord restore peace
to Europe.
*For I meditate the peace of Europe amongst family bickerings and
domestic jars.*

Let Zuar rejoice with the Guinea Hen—The Lord add to his mercies
in the WEST!
*For the HOST is in the WEST—the Lord make us thankful unto
salvation.*

Let Chesed rejoice with Strepsiceros, whose weapons are the
  ornaments of his peace.
*For I preach the very GOSPEL of CHRIST without comment and with
  this weapon shall I slay envy.*

Let Hagar rejoice with Gnesion, who is the right sort of eagle, and
  towers the highest.
For I bless God in the rising generation, which is on my side.

Let Libni rejoice with the Redshank, who migrates not but is
  translated to the upper regions.
*For I have translated in the charity, which makes things better and
  I shall be translated myself at the last.*

Let Nahshon rejoice with the Seabreese, the Lord gives the sailors of
  his Spirit.
*For he that walked upon the sea, hath prepared the floods with the
  Gospel of peace.*

Let Helon rejoice with the Woodpecker—the Lord encourage the
  propagation of trees!
*For the merciful man is merciful to his beast, and to the trees that give
  them shelter.*

Let Amos rejoice with the Coote—prepare to meet thy God, O Israel.
*For he hath turned the shadow of death into the morning, the Lord is
  his name.*

Let Ephah rejoice with Buprestis, the Lord endue us with temperance
  and humanity, till every cow have her mate!
*For I am come home again, but there is nobody to kill the calf or to pay
  the music.*

Let Sarah rejoice with the Redwing, whose harvest is in the frost and
  snow.
*For the hour of my felicity, like the womb of Sarah, shall come at the
  latter end.*

Let Rebekah rejoice with Iynx, who holds his head on one side to
  deceive the adversary.
*For I should have avail'd myself of waggery, had not malice been
  multitudinous.*

Let Shuah rejoice with Boa, which is the vocal serpent.
For there are still serpents that can speak—God bless my head, my heart and my heel.

Let Ehud rejoice with Onocrotalus, whose braying is for the glory of God, because he makes the best music in his power.
For I bless God that I am of the same seed as Ehud, Mutius Scaevola, and Colonel Draper.

Let Shamgar rejoice with Otis, who looks about him for the glory of God, and sees the horizon complete at once.
For the word of God is a sword on my side—no matter what other weapon a stick or a straw.

Let Bohan rejoice with the Scythian Stag—he is beef and breeches against want and nakedness.
For I have adventured myself in the name of the Lord, and he hath mark'd me for his own.

Let Achsah rejoice with the Pigeon who is an antidote to malignity and will carry a letter.
For I bless God for the Postmaster general and all conveyancers of letters under his care especially Allen and Shelvock.

Let Tohu rejoice with the Grouse—the Lord further the cultivating of heaths and the peopling of deserts.
For my grounds in New Canaan shall infinitely compensate for the flats and mains of Staindrop Moor.

Let Hillel rejoice with Ammodytes, whose colour is deceitful and he plots against the pilgrim's feet.
For the praise of God can give to a mute fish the notes of a nightingale.

Let Eli rejoice with Leucon—he is an honest fellow, which is a rarity.
For I have seen the White Raven and Thomas Hall of Willingham and am my self a greater curiosity than both.

Let Jemuel rejoice with Charadrius, who is from the HEIGHT and the sight of him is good for the jaundice.
For I look up to heaven which is my prospect to escape envy by surmounting it.

. . .

For I will consider my Cat Jeoffry.

For he is the servant of the Living God duly and daily serving him.

For at the first glance of the glory of God in the East he worships in his way.

For is this done by wreathing his body seven times round with elegant quickness.

For then he leaps up to catch the musk, which is the blessing of God upon his prayer.

For he rolls upon prank to work it in.

For having done duty and received blessing he begins to consider himself.

For this he performs in ten degrees.

For first he looks upon his fore-paws to see if they are clean.

For secondly he kicks up behind to clear away there.

For thirdly he works it upon stretch with the fore-paws extended.

For fourthly he sharpens his paws by wood.

For fifthly he washes himself.

For sixthly he rolls upon wash.

For seventhly he fleas himself, that he may not be interrupted upon the beat.

For eighthly he rubs himself against a post.

For ninthly he looks up for his instructions.

For tenthly he goes in quest of food.

For having consider'd God and himself he will consider his neighbour.

For if he meets another cat he will kiss her in kindness.

For when he takes his prey he plays with it to give it chance.

For one mouse in seven escapes by his dallying.

For when his day's work is done his business more properly begins.

For he keeps the Lord's watch in the night against the adversary.

For he counteracts the powers of darkness by his electrical skin and glaring eyes.

For he counteracts the Devil, who is death, by brisking about the life.

For in his morning orisons he loves the sun and the sun loves him.

For he is of the tribe of Tiger.

For the Cherub Cat is a term of the Angel Tiger.

For he has the subtlety and hissing of a serpent, which in goodness he suppresses.

For he will not do destruction, if he is well-fed, neither will he spit without provocation.

For he purrs in thankfulness, when God tells him he's a good Cat.

For he is an instrument for the children to learn benevolence upon.

For every house is incomplete without him and a blessing is lacking in the spirit.

For the Lord commanded Moses concerning the cats at the departure of the Children of Israel from Egypt.

For every family had one cat at least in the bag.

For the English Cats are the best in Europe.

For he is the cleanest in the use of his fore-paws of any quadrupede.

For the dexterity of his defence is an instance of the love of God to him exceedingly.

For he is the quickest to his mark of any creature.

For he is tenacious of his point.

For he is a mixture of gravity and waggery.

For he knows that God is his Saviour.

For there is nothing sweeter than his peace when at rest.

For there is nothing brisker than his life when in motion.

For he is of the Lord's poor and so indeed is he called by benevolence perpetually—Poor Jeoffry! poor Jeoffry! the rat has bit thy throat.

For I bless the name of the Lord Jesus that Jeoffry is better.

For the divine spirit comes about his body to sustain it in complete cat.

For his tongue is exceeding pure so that it has in purity what it wants in music.

For he is docile and can learn certain things.

For he can set up with gravity which is patience upon approbation.

For he can fetch and carry, which is patience in employment.

For he can jump over a stick which is patience upon proof positive.

For he can spraggle upon waggle at the word of command.

For he can jump from an eminence into his master's bosom.

For he can catch the cork and toss it again.

For he is hated by the hypocrite and miser.

For the former is afraid of detection.

For the latter refuses the charge.

For he camels his back to bear the first notion of business.

For he is good to think on, if a man would express himself neatly.

For he made a great figure in Egypt for his signal services.

For he killed the Ichneumon-rat very pernicious by land.

For his ears are so acute that they sting again.

For from this proceeds the passing quickness of his attention.

For by stroking of him I have found out electricity.

For I perceived God's light about him both wax and fire.

For the Electrical fire is the spiritual substance, which God sends from heaven to sustain the bodies both of man and beast.

For God has blessed him in the variety of his movements.
For, tho' he cannot fly, he is an excellent clamberer.
For his motions upon the face of the earth are more than any other
  quadrupede.
For he can tread to all the measures upon the music.
For he can swim for life.
For he can creep.

Thomas Warton

(1728–1790)

from "The Pleasures of Melancholy"

Mother of musings, Contemplation sage,
Whose grotto stands upon the topmost rock
Of Teneriff: 'mid the tempestuous night,
On which, in calmest meditation held,
Thou hear'st with howling winds the beating rain
And drifting hail descend; or if the skies
Unclouded shine, and thro' the blue serene
Pale Cynthia rolls her silver-axled car,
Whence gazing stedfast on the spangled vault
Raptur'd thou sit'st, while murmurs indistinct
Of distant billows sooth thy pensive ear
With hoarse and hollow sounds; secure, self-blest,
There oft thou listen'st to the wild uproar
Of fleets encount'ring, that in whispers low
Ascends the rocky summit, where thou dwell'st
Remote from man, conversing with the spheres!
O lead me, queen sublime, to solemn glooms
Congenial with my soul; to cheerless shades,
To ruin'd seats, or twilight cells and bow'rs,
Where thoughtful Melancholy loves to muse,
Her fav'rite midnight haunts. The laughing scenes
Of purple Spring, where all the wanton train
Of Smiles and Graces seem to lead the dance
In sportive round, while from their hands they show'r
Ambrosial blooms and flow'rs, no longer charm;
Tempe, no more I court thy balmy breeze,
Adieu green vales! ye broider'd meads, adieu!

. . .

Thro' Pope's soft song tho' all the Graces breathe,
And happiest art adorn his Attic page;
Yet does my mind with sweeter transport glow,
As at the root of mossy trunk reclin'd,

In magic Spenser's wildly-warbled song
I see deserted Una wander wide
Thro' wasteful solitudes, and lurid heaths
Weary, forlorn; than when the fated fair,
Upon the bosom bright of silver Thames,
Launches in all the lustre of brocade,
Amid the splendors of the laughing Sun.
The gay description palls upon the sense,
And coldly strikes the mind with feeble bliss.

Ye Youths of Albion's beauty-blooming isle,
Whose brows have worn the wreath of luckless love,
Is there a pleasure like the pensive mood,
Whose magic wont to sooth your soften'd souls?
O tell how rapturous the joy, to melt
To Melody's assuasive voice; to bend
Th'uncertain step along the midnight mead,
And pour your sorrows to the pitying moon,
By many a slow trill from the bird of woe
Oft interrupted; in embowering woods
By darksome brook to muse, and there forget
The solemn dulness of the tedious world,
While Fancy grasps the visionary fair:
And now no more th'abstracted ear attends
The water's murm'ring lapse, th'entranced eye
Pierces no longer thro' th'extended rows
Of thick-rang'd trees; 'till haply from the depth
The woodman's stroke, or distant-tinkling team,
Or heifer rustling thro' the brake alarms
Th'illuded sense, and mars the golden dream.
These are delights that absence drear has made
Familiar to my soul, e'er since the form
Of young Sapphira, beauteous as the Spring,
When from her vi'let-woven couch awak'd
By frolic Zephyr's hand, her tender cheek
Graceful she lifts, and blushing from her bow'r,
Issues to cloath in gladsome-glist'ring green
The genial globe, first met my dazzled sight:
These are delights unknown to minds profane,
And which alone the pensive soul can taste.

· · ·

113

William Cowper

(1731–1800)

Lines Written During a Period of Insanity

Hatred and vengence—my eternal portion
Scarce can endure delay of execution—
Wait with impatient readiness to seize my
Soul in a moment.

Damned below Judas; more abhorred than he was,
Who for a few pence sold his holy Master!
Twice betrayed, Jesus me, the last delinquent,
Deems the profanest.

Man disavows, and Deity disowns me:
Hell might afford my miseries a shelter;
Therefore Hell keeps her ever-hungry mouths all
Bolted against me.

Hard lot! encompassed with a thousand dangers;
Weary, faint, trembling with a thousand terrors,
I'm called, if vanquished, to receive a sentence
Worse than Abiram's.

Him the vindictive rod of angry Justice
Sent quick and howling to the centre headlong;
I, fed with judgment, in a fleshy tomb am
Buried above ground.

The Shrubbery, Written in a Time of Affliction

　　　Oh happy shades—to me unblest!
Friendly to peace, but not to me!
How ill the scene that offers rest,
And heart that cannot rest, agree!

This glassy stream, that spreading pine
Those alders quiv'ring to the breeze,
Might sooth a soul less hurt than mine,
And please, if any thing could please.

But fix'd unalterable care
Foregoes not what she feels within,
Shows the same sadness ev'rywhere,
And slights the season and the scene.

For all that pleas'd in wood or lawn,
While peace possess'd these silent bow'rs,
Her animating smile withdrawn,
Has lost its beauties and its pow'rs.

The saint or moralist should tread
This moss-grown alley, musing, slow;
They seek, like me, the secret shade,
But not, like me, to nourish woe!

Me fruitful scenes and prospects waste
Alike admonish not to roam;
These tell me of enjoyments past,
And those of sorrows yet to come.

Anonymous

(published 1733)

A Receipt to Cure a Love Fit

Tie one end of a rope fast over a beam,
And make a slip-noose at the other extreme;
Then just underneath let a cricket be set,
On which let the lover most manfully get;
Then over his head let the snecket be got,
And under one ear be well settled the knot.
The cricket kicked down, let him take a fair swing;
And leave all the rest of the work to the string.

Robert Fergusson

(1750–1774)

Ode to Disappointment

I

Thou joyless fiend, life's constant foe,
Sad *source* of care and *spring* of woe,
   Soft pleasure's hard controul;
Her gayest haunts for ever nigh,
Stern mistress of the secret sigh,
   That swells the murm'ring soul.

II

Why haunt'st thou me thro' desart drear?
With grief-swoln sounds why wound my ear,
   Denied to *pity's* aid?
Thy visage wan did e'er I woo,
Or at thy feet in homage bow,
   Or court thy sullen shade.

III

Even now enchanted scenes abound,
Elysian glories strew the ground,
   To lure th'astonish'd eyes;
Now *Horrors, Hell*, and *Furies* reign,
And desolate the fairy scene
   Of all its gay disguise.

IV

The passions, at thy urgent call,
Our *reasons* and our *sense* inthrall
   In frenzy's fetters strong.
And now *despair* with lurid eye
Doth meagre *poverty* discry,
   Subdu'd by famine long.

V

The lover flies the haunts of day,
In gloomy woods and wilds to stray,
   There shuns his *Jessy's* scorn;
Sad sisters of the sighing grove
Attune their lyres to hapless love,
   Dejected and forlorn.

VI

Yet *hope* undaunted wears thy *chain*,
And *smiles* amidst the growing *pain*,
   Nor fears thy sad dismay;
Unaw'd by power her fancy flies
From earth's dim *orb* to purer skies,
   Realms of endless *day*.

Anonymous

(published 1751)

Strip Me Naked, or Royal Gin for Ever. A Picture

I must, I will have gin!–that skillet take,
Pawn it.—No more I'll roast, or boil or bake.
This juice immortal will each want supply;
Starve on, ye brats! So I but bung my eye.
Starve? No! This gin ev'n mother's milk excels,
Paints the pale cheeks, and hunger's darts repels.
The skillet's pawned already? Take this cap;
Round my bare head I'll yon brown paper wrap.
Ha! Half my petticoat was torn away
By dogs (I fancy) as I maudlin lay.
How the wind whistles through each broken pane!
Through the wide-yawning roof how pours the rain!
My bedstead's cracked; the table goes hip-hop.—
But see! The gin! Come, come, thou cordial drop!
Thou sovereign balsam to my longing heart!
Thou husband, children, all! We must not part!

Drinks   Delicious! O! Down the red lane it goes;
Now I'm a queen, and trample on my woes.
Inspired by gin, I'm ready for the road;
Could shoot my man, or fire the King's abode.
Ha! My brain's cracked.—The room turns round and round;
Down drop the platters, pans: I'm on the ground.
My tattered gown slips from me.—What care I?
I was born naked, and I'll naked die.

Thomas Chatterton

(1752–1770)

Sunday, A Fragment

Hervenis, harping on the hackneyed text,
By disquisitions is so sore perplexed,
He stammers,—instantaneously is drawn
A bordered piece of inspiration-lawn,
Which being thrice unto his nose applied,
Into his pineal gland the vapours glide;
And now again we hear the doctor roar
On subjects he dissected thrice before.
I own at church I very seldom pray,
For vicars, strangers to devotion, bray.
Sermons, though flowing from the sacred lawn,
Are flimsy wires from reason's ingot drawn;
And, to confess the truth, another cause
My every prayer and adoration draws:
In all the glaring tinctures of the bow,
The ladies front me in celestial row.
(Though, when black melancholy damps my joys,
I call them nature's trifles, airy toys;
Yet when the goddess Reason guides the strain,
I think them, what they are, a heavenly train.)
The amorous rolling, the black sparkling eye,
The gentle hazel, and the optic sly;
The easy shape, the panting semi-globes,
The frankness which each latent charm disrobes;
The melting passions, and the sweet severe,
The easy amble, the majestic air;
The tapering waist, the silver-mantled arms,
All is one vast variety of charms.
Say, who but sages stretched beyond their span,
Italian singers, or an unmanned man,
Can see Elysium spread upon their brow,
And to a drowsy curate's sermon bow?

If (but 'tis seldom) no fair female face
Attracts my notice by some glowing grace,
Around the monuments I cast my eyes,
And see absurdities and nonsense rise.
Here rueful-visaged angels seem to tell,
With weeping eyes, a soul is gone to hell;
There a child's head, supported by duck's wings,
With toothless mouth a hallelujah sings:
In funeral pile eternal marble burns,
And a good Christian seems to sleep in urns.
A self-drawn curtain bids the reader see
An honourable Welchman's pedigree;
A rock of porphyry darkens half the place,
And virtues blubber with no awkward grace;
Yet, strange to tell, in all the dreary gloom
That makes the sacred honours of the tomb,
No quartered coats above the base appear,
No battered arms, or golden corsets there.

John Codrington Bampfylde

(1754–1796)

On a Frightful Dream

This morn ere yet had rung the matin peal,
   The cursed Merlin, with his potent spell,
   Aggrieved me sore, and from his wizard cell,
   (First fixing on mine eyes a magic seal)
Millions of ghosts and shadowy shapes let steal;
   Who, swarming round my couch, with horrid yell,
   Chattered and mocked, as though from deepest Hell
   They had escaped.—I oft, with fervent zeal,
Essayed, and prayer, to mar the enchanter's power.
   In vain for thicker still the crew came on,
   And now had weighed me down, but that the day
Appeared, and Phoebus, from his eastern tower,
   With new-tricked beam, like truth immortal, shone,
   And chased the visionary forms away.

William Blake

(1757–1827)

"My Spectre around me night and day"

My Spectre around me night and
Like a wild beast guards my way;
My Emanation far within
Weeps incessantly for my sin.

A fathomless and boundless deep,
There we wander, there we weep;
On the hungry craving wind
My Spectre follows thee behind.

He scents thy footsteps in the snow,
Wheresoever thou dost go,
Thro' the wintry hail and rain.
When wilt thou return again?

Dost thou not in pride and scorn
Fill with tempests all my morn,
And with jealousies and fears
Fill my pleasant nights with tears?

Seven of my sweet loves thy knife
Has bereavèd of their life.
Their marble tombs I built with tears,
And with cold and shuddering fears.

Seven more loves weep night and day
Round the tombs where my loves lay,
And seven more loves attend each night
Around my couch with torches bright.

And seven more loves in my bed
Crown with wine my mournful head,

Pitying and forgiving all
Thy transgressions great and small.

When wilt thou return and view
My loves, and them to life renew?
When wilt thou return and live?
When wilt thou pity as I forgive?

O'er my sins thou sit and moan:
Hast thou no sins of thy own?
O'er my sins thou sit and weep,
And lull thy own sins fast asleep.

What transgressions I commit
Are for thy transgressions fit.
They thy harlots, thou their slave;
And my bed becomes their grave.

Never, never, I return:
Still for victory I burn.
Living, thee alone I'll have;
And when dead I'll be thy grave.

Thro' the Heaven and Earth and Hell
Thou shalt never, never quell:
I will fly and thou pursue:
Night and morn the flight renew.

Poor, pale, pitiable form
That I follow in a storm;
Iron tears and groans of lead
Bind around my aching head.

Till I turn from Female love
And root up the Infernal Grove,
I shall never worthy be
To step into Eternity.

And, to end thy cruel mocks,
Annihilate thee on the rocks,
And another form create
To be subservient to my fate.

Let us agree to give up love,
And root up the Infernal Grove;
Then shall we return and see
The worlds of happy Eternity.

And throughout all Eternity
I forgive you, you forgive me.
As our dear Redeemer said:
"This the Wine, and this the Bread."

To Mr. Butts, Gr. Marlborough St., London; from *Letters, A Selection*

O why was I born with a different face
Why was I not born like the rest of my race
When I look each one starts! when I speak I offend
Then I'm silent & passive & lose every Friend

Then my verse I dishonour. My pictures despise
My person degrade & my temper chastise
And the pen is my terror, the pencil my shame
All my Talents I bury, and dead is my Fame

I am either too low or too highly prizd
When Elate I am Envy'd, When Meek I'm despis'd

Mary

Sweet Mary the first time she ever was there
Came into the Ball room among the Fair

The young Men & Maidens around her throng
And these are the words upon every tongue

An Angel is here from the heavenly Climes
Or again does return the Golden times
Her eyes outshine every brilliant ray
She opens her lips tis the Month of May

Mary moves in soft beauty & conscious delight
To augment with sweet smiles all the joys of the Night
Nor once blushes to own to the rest of the Fair
That sweet Love & Beauty are worthy our care

In the Morning the Villagers rose with delight
And repeated with pleasure the joys of the night
And Mary arose among Friends to be free
But no Friend from henceforward thou Mary shalt see

Some said she was proud some calld her a whore
And some when she passed by shut to the door
A damp cold came oer her her blushes all fled
Her lillies & roses are blighted & shed

O why was I born with a different Face
Why was I not born like this Envious Race
Why did Heaven adorn me with bountiful hand
And then set me down in an envious Land

To be weak as a Lamb & smooth as a dove
And not to raise Envy is calld Christian Love
But if you raise Envy your Merits to blame
For planting such spite in the weak & the tame

I will humble my Beauty I will not dress fine
I will keep from the Ball & my Eyes shall not shine
And if any Girls Lover forsakes her for me
I'll refuse him my hand & from Envy be free

She went out in Morning attird plain & neat
Proud Marys gone Mad said the Child in the Street
She went out in Morning in plain neat attire
And came home in Evening bespatterd with mire

126

She trembled & wept sitting on the Bed side
She forgot it was Night & she trembled & cried
She forgot it was Night she forgot it was Morn
Her soft Memory imprinted with Faces of Scorn

With Faces of Scorn & with Eyes of disdain
Like foul Fiends inhabiting Marys mild Brain
She remembers no Face like the Human Divine
All Faces have Envy sweet Mary but thine

And thine is a Face of sweet Love in Despair
And thine is a Face of mild sorrow & care
And thine is a Face of wild terror & fear
That shall never be quiet till laid on its bier

Mad Song

   The wild winds
And the night is a-cold;
Come hither, Sleep,
And my griefs infold:
But lo! the morning peeps
Over the eastern steeps,
And the rustling birds of dawn
The earth do scorn.

Lo! to the vault
Of paved heaven,
With sorrow fraught
My notes are driven:
They strike the ear of night,
Make weep the eyes of day;
They make mad the roaring winds,
And with tempests play.

Like a fiend in a cloud,
With howling woe,
After night I do crowd,
And with night will go;
I turn my back to the east,
From whence comforts have increas'd;
For light doth seize my brain
With frantic pain.

Robert Bloomfield

(1766–1823)

from "The Farmer's Boy"

. . .

Hither at times, with cheerfulness of soul,
Sweet *village Maids* from neighbouring hamlets stroll,
That like the light-heel'd does o'er lawns that rove,
Look shyly curious; rip'ning into love;
For love's their errand: hence the tints that glow
On either cheek, a heighten'd lustre know:
When, conscious of their charms, e'en Age looks sly,
And rapture beams from Youth's observant eye.

The pride of such a party, Nature's pride
Was lovely **Ann**, who innocently try'd,
With hat of airy shape and ribbons gay,
Love to inspire, and stand in Hymen's way
But, ere her *twentieth* Summer could expand,
Or youth was render'd happy with her hand,
Her mind's serenity, her peace was gone,
Her eye grew languid, and she wept alone

Yet causeless seem'd her grief; for quick restrain'd,
Mirth follow'd loud; or indignation reign'd:
Whims wild and simple led her from her home,
The heath, the common, or the fields to roam:
Terror and Joy alternate rul'd her hours;
Now blithe she sung, and gather'd useless flow'rs;
Now pluck'd a tender twig from ev'ry bough,
To whip the hov'ring demons from her brow.
Ill-fated Maid! thy guiding spark is fled,
And lasting wretchedness awaits thy bed—
Thy bed of straw! for mark, where even now
O'er their lost child afflicted parents bow;
Their woe she knows not, but perversely coy,

Inverted customs yield her sullen joy;
Her midnight meals in secrecy she takes,
Low mutt'ring to the moon, that rising breaks
Thro' night's dark gloom:—oh how much more forlorn
Her night, that knows of no returning morn!—

Slow from the threshold, once her infant seat,
O'er the cold earth she crawls to her retreat;
Quitting the cot's warm walls, unhous'd to lie,
Or share the swine's impure and narrow sty;
The damp night air her shiv'ring limbs assails;
In dreams she moans, and fancied wrongs bewails.
When morning wakes, none earlier rous'd than she,
When pendent drops fall glitt'ring from the tree;
But nought her rayless melancholy cheers,
Or sooths her breast, or stops her streaming tears.

Her matted locks unornamented flow;
Clasping her knees, and waving to and fro;—
Her head bow'd down, her faded cheek to hide;—
A piteous mourner by the pathway side.
Some tufted molehill through the livelong day
She calls her throne; there weeps her life away:
And oft the gaily-passing stranger stays
His well-tim'd step, and takes a silent gaze,

Till sympathetic drops unbidden start,
And pangs quick springing muster round his heart;
And soft he treads with other gazers round,
And fain would catch her sorrows' plaintive sound:
One word alone is all that strikes the ear,
One short, pathetic, simple word,—"*Oh dear!*"
A thousand times repeated to the wind,
That wafts the sigh, but leaves the pang behind!

. . .

Samuel Taylor Coleridge

(1772–1834)

The Suicide's Argument

Ere the birth of my life, if I wished it or no
No question was asked me—it could not be so!
If the life was the question, a thing sent to try
And to live on be YES; what can NO be? to die.

Nature's Answer:

Is't returned, as 'twas sent? Is't no worse for the wear?
Think first, what you ARE! Call to mind what you WERE!
I gave you innocence, I gave you hope,
Gave health, and genius, and an ample scope,
Return you me guilt, lethargy, despair?
Make out the invent'ry; inspect, compare!
Then die—if die you dare!

The Pains of Sleep

Ere on my bed my limbs I lay,
It hath not been my use to pray
With moving lips or bended knees;
But silently, by slow degrees,
My spirit I to Love compose,
In humble trust mine eye-lids close,
With reverential resignation,
No wish conceived, no thought exprest,
Only a sense of supplication;

A sense o'er all my soul imprest
That I am weak, yet not unblest,
Since in me, round me, every where
Eternal Strength and Wisdom are.

But yester-night I prayed aloud
In anguish and in agony,
Up-starting from the fiendish crowd
Of shapes and thoughts that tortured me:
A lurid light, a trampling throng,
Sense of intolerable wrong,
And whom I scorned, those only strong!
Thirst of revenge, the powerless will
Still baffled, and yet burning still!
Desire with loathing strangely mixed
On wild or hateful objects fixed.
Fantastic passions! maddening brawl!
And shame and terror over all!
Deeds to be hid which were not hid,
Which all confused I could not know
Whether I suffered, or I did:
For all seemed guilt, remorse or woe,
My own or others still the same
Life-stifling fear, soul-stifling shame.

So two nights passed: the night's dismay
Saddened and stunned the coming day.
Sleep, the wide blessing, seemed to me
Distemper's worst calamity.
The third night, when my own loud scream
Had waked me from the fiendish dream,
O'ercome with sufferings strange and wild,
I wept as I had been a child;
And having thus by tears subdued
My anguish to a milder mood,
Such punishments, I said, were due
To natures deepliest stained with sin,—
For aye entempesting anew
The unfathomable hell within,
The horror of their deeds to view,
To know and loathe, yet wish and do!

Such griefs with such men well agree,
But wherefore, wherefore fall on me?
To be beloved is all I need,
And whom I love, I love indeed.

❧

. . .

II
A grief without a pang, void, dark, and drear,
A stifled, drowsy, unimpassioned grief,
Which finds no natural outlet, no relief,
    In word, or sigh, or tear—
O Lady! in this wan and heartless mood,
To other thoughts by yonder throstle woo'd,
All this long eve, so balmy and serene,
Have I been gazing on the western sky,
And its peculiar tint of yellow green:
And still I gaze—and with how blank an eye!
And those thin clouds above, in flakes and bars,
That give away their motion to the stars;
Those stars, that glide behind them or between,
Now sparkling, now bedimmed, but always seen:
Yon crescent Moon, as fixed as if it grew
In its own cloudless, starless lake of blue;
I see them all so excellently fair,
I see, not feel, how beautiful they are!

III
    My genial spirits fail;
    And what can these avail
To lift the smothering weight from off my breast?
    It were a vain endeavour,
    Though I should gaze for ever
On that green light that lingers in the west:

I may not hope from outward forms to win
The passion and the life, whose fountains are within.

. . .

VI

There was a time when, though my path was rough,
This joy within me dallied with distress,
And all misfortunes were but as the stuff
Whence Fancy made me dreams of happiness:
For hope grew round me, like the twining vine,
And fruits, and foliage, not my own, seemed mine.
But now afflictions bow me down to earth:
Nor care I that they rob me of my mirth;
        But oh! each visitation
Suspends what nature gave me at my birth,
My shaping spirit of Imagination.
For not to think of what I needs must feel,
But to be still and patient, all I can;
And haply by abstruse research to steal
From my own nature all the natural man—
This was my sole resource, my only plan:
Till that which suits a part infects the whole,
And now is almost grown the habit of my soul.

VII

Hence, viper thoughts, that coil around my mind,
        Reality's dark dream!
I turn from you, and listen to the wind,
Which long has raved unnoticed. What a scream
Of agony by torture lengthened out
That lute sent forth! Thou Wind, that rav'st without,
Bare crag, or mountain-tairn, or blasted tree,
Or pine-grove whither woodman never clomb,
Or lonely house, long held the witches' home,
Methinks were fitter instruments for thee,
Mad Lutanist! who in this month of showers,
Of dark-brown gardens, and of peeping flowers,
Mak'st Devils' yule, with worse than wintry song,
The blossoms, buds, and timorous leaves among.
Thou Actor, perfect in all tragic sounds!
Thou mighty Poet, e'en to frenzy bold!

What tell'st thou now about?
'Tis of the rushing of an host in rout,
With groans, of trampled men, with smarting wounds—
At once they groan with pain, and shudder with the cold!

. . .

George Gordon, Lord Byron

(1788–1824)

from "The Lament of Tasso"

. . .

I

Long years!—It tries the thrilling frame to bear
And eagle-spirit of a Child of Song—
Long years of outrage—calumny—and wrong;
Imputed madness, prisoned solitude,
And the Mind's canker in its savage mood,
When the impatient thirst of light and air
Parches the heart; and the abhorred grate,
Marring the sunbeams with its hideous shade,
Works through the throbbing eyeball to the brain,
With a hot sense of heaviness and pain;
And bare, at once, Captivity displayed
Stands scoffing through the never-opened gate,
Which nothing through its bars admits, save day,
And tasteless food, which I have eat alone
Till its unsocial bitterness is gone;
And I can banquest like a beast of prey,
Sullen and lonely, couching in the cave
Which is my lair, and—it may be—my grave.
All this hath somewhat worn me, and may wear,
But must be borne. I stoop not to despair;
For I have battled with mine agony,
And made me wings wherewith to overfly
The narrow circus of my dungeon wall . . .

. . .

III

Above me, hark! the long and maniac cry
Of minds and bodies in captivity.
And hark! the lash and the increasing howl,
And the half-inarticulate blasphemy!

136

There be some here with worse than frenzy foul,
Some who do still goad on the o'er-laboured mind,
And dim the little light that's left behind
With needless torture, as their tyrant Will
Is wound up to the lust of doing ill:
With these and with their victims am I classed,
'Mid sounds and sights like these long years have passed;
'Mid sights and sounds like these my life may close:
So let it be—for then I shall repose.

　　IV
I have been patient, let me be so yet;
I had forgotten half I would forget,
But it revives—Oh! would it were my lot
To be forgetful as I am forgot!—
Feel I not wroth with those who bade me
In this vast Lazar-house of many woes?
Where laughter is not mirth, nor thought the mind,
Nor words a language, nor ev'n men mankind;
Where cries reply to curses, shrieks to blows,
And each is tortured in his separate hell—
For we are crowded in our solitudes—
Many, but each divided by the wall,
Which echoes Madness in her babbling moods;
While all can hear, non heed his neighbour's call—
None! save that One, the veriest wretch of all,
Who was not made to be the mate of these,
Nor bound between Distraction and Disease,
Feel I not wroth with those who placed me here?
Who have debased me in the minds of men,
Debarring me the usage of my own,
Blighting my life in best of its career,
Branding my thoughts as things to shun and fear?

· · ·

Percy Bysshe Shelley

(1792–1822)

Stanzas Written in Dejection Near Naples

The sun is warm, the sky is clear,
The waves are dancing fast and bright,
Blue isles and snowy mountains wear
The purple noon's transparent might,
The breath of the moist earth is light,
Around its unexpanded buds;
Like many a voice of one delight
The winds, the birds, the ocean floods,
The city's voice itself, is soft like Solitude's.

I see the deep's untrampled floor
With green and purple seaweeds strown;
I see the waves upon the shore,
Like light dissolved in star-showers, thrown:
I sit upon the sands alone,—
The lightning of the noontide ocean
Is flashing round me, and a tone
Arises from its measured motion,
How sweet! did any heart now share in my emotion.

Alas! I have nor hope nor health,
Nor peace within nor calm around,
Nor that content surpassing wealth
The sage in meditation found,
And walked with inward glory crowned—
Nor fame, nor power, nor love, nor leisure,
Others I see whom these surround—
Smiling they live, and call life pleasure;—
To me that cup has been dealt in another measure.

Yet now despair itself is mild,
Even as the winds and waters are;

I could lie down like a tired child,
And weep away the life of care
Which I have born and yet must bear,
Till death like sleep might steal on me,
And I might feel in the warm air
My cheek grow cold, and hear the sea
Breathe o'er my dying brain its last monotony.

Some might lament that I were cold,
As I, when this sweet day is gone,
Which my lost heart, too soon grown old,
Insults with this untimely moan;
They might lament—for I am one
Whom men love not,—and yet regret,
Unlike this day, which, when the sun
Shall on its stainless glory set,
Will linger, though enjoyed, like joy in memory yet.

John Clare

(1793–1864)

I Am

I am—yet what I am, none cares or knows;
   My friends forsake me like a memory lost:—
I am the self-consumer of my woes;—
   They rise and vanish in oblivion's host,
Like shadows in love's frenzied stifled throes:—
And yet I am, and live—like vapours tost

Into the nothingness of scorn and noise,—
   Into the living sea of waking dreams,
Where there is neither sense of life or joys,
   But the vast shipwreck of my lifes esteems;
Even the dearest, that I love the best
Are strange—nay, rather stranger than the rest.

I long for scenes, where man hath never trod
   A place where woman never smiled or wept
There to abide with my Creator, God;
   And sleep as I in childhood, sweetly slept,
Untroubling, and untroubled where I lie,
The grass below—above the vaulted sky.

Sonnet: I Am

I feel I am;—I only know I am,
And plod upon the earth, as dull and void:
Earth's prison chilled my body with its dram

Of dullness, and my soaring thoughts destroyed,
I fled to solitudes from passions dream,
But strife persued—I only know, I am,
I was a being created in the race
Of men disdaining bounds of place and time:—
A spirit that could travel o'er the space
Of earth and heaven,—like a thought sublime,
Tracing creation, like my maker, free,—
A soul unshackled—like eternity,
Spurning earth's vain and soul debasing thrall
But now I only know I am,—that's all.

The Ruins of Despair

Yon mouldering wall compos'd of nought but mud
(Which has for ages in that manner stood)
Is rightly stil'd the 'Ruins of Despair'
For nought but wretchedness assembles there
All sons of grief and daughters of despair
Within that hut;—but how can life live there?
Thats strange indeed,—while these old walls of mud
('Which has for ages in that manner stood')
Keeps daily mouldering in a lost decay
Leaning on props that want themselves a stay!
Well may those wrankling nettles thrive and grow
So duley water'd with the tears of woe,
—Lo on the floor with gulling holes o'erspread
Their wretched feet betray a shooles tread:—
The 'Ruins' covering nought but loose-laid straw
Which winds blow off and leave a frequent flaw
There snows drive in upon the wretches head
There hasty rains a threatn'd deluge shed
Thrice wretched wretched 'Ruins of despair'
What griefs are thine.—O 'how can life live there?'
—A rag-stuft hole,—where bits of Lead remain

Proof of what was,—but now without a pane
A roof unceal'd displays the rafters bare
Here dangling straws and cobwebs dropping there
No white-wash'd walls to pictur'd taste incline
Instead of pictures threatn'd carvings shine
The dismal harth is nothing but a hole
To wood a stranger and the same to coal
Light straw and rubbish make their sorry fires
Kindl'd no quicker than the flame expires
Instead of chairs great stones bedeck the ground
(Rough seats indeed!)—and closley raing'd around
On these the wretched tribe spend half their days
Dythering and weeping oer the dying blaze
A blaze that does more paint than heat supply
Tingeing their faces with a smoaky dye.—
No shelves no Cubboards no convieneience there
'T'was plan'd in grief and finish'd with despair
They make their shelves and cubboards on the floor
In a dark hole behind the broken door
There an old pitcher broke beyond excuse
(For wants consceald by them is little use)
Stands with the filthy shadow of a pan
Filthy and nausious,—O!—what being—can
Endure!—Grief searching muse give oer
On such a dismal scene essay no more
Stay thy too curious search,—forbear,—forbear,
No more describe the 'Ruins of Despair!
O if the sorrows which true love inspires
In heavens eye could ere compasion find
O give ye gods my hearts supreme desire
& teach my angle myra to be kind
The lovly charmer she is all to me
My utmost hopes—the all my heart desires
& O beneath her scorn my pleasure flees
& all my wishes & my hopes expires
For her my Youth & vigour pines away
For her black sadnes truns my day to night
And by her Frown my chill soul shrinks away
And life itself grows hateful to my sight
Adieu the pleasures which I once posest
Those tastles charms that gave deligt & ease
The charms of her supplanted all the rest

& those posesd by her alone can please
In vain all pleasures art & nature yields
My sickning soul their sweetest pastimes shun
& like the blighted blossom of the fields
Sickens & dies beneath the brightest sun
Possesd of her the remedy is sure
All heaven is present when the charmers there
Denyd of her theres nought admits a cure
Absence is hell—I perish in despair

To Melancholy

Come maiden sad—of sorrows and of sighs
Pale melancholy! with the downcast look,
Come when the dewy eve the landscape dyes:
The church yard yew we'll pass, and gurgling brook,
And see the snow white moth, on stilly breeze,
Dance by the spinney hedge, & through the leaves.
While the dull visions trouble, and deceives
Thy soul with troubles all thine own:
The stilly eve, thy secret woe receives.
Maiden thou'rt like the church yards mossy stone,
Thou readest thy troubles to the world unknown,
Thy kind face soothes all sorrow save thine own.

Song

& when I'm weary of my care
& when I wish to loose a pain
Gi me an easy elbow chair

& bottle full of wine to drain
& gi me two three croney men
Wi song & fun my joys to crown
Some hearty oddlings like my sen
The choicest cocks about the town

& round the sparkling glasses put
& each one take a hearty pull
& like brave boy sit foot to foot
Till sorrows got his belly full
& drink till each can keep his seat
Then held up by his fellow man
Some two three bouts agen repeat
& drown old sorrow if we can

Nor from his bumpers none decline
Till one wi in his seat can keep
Till griefs near chokd chin deep in wine
& sorrows dozd to dream less sleep

& who fails first shall pay his fee
& whos a sinner wine to spill
The judgment on his sins shall be
A bottle from his purse to fill
So drink brave boys till care & pain
To see their weapons usless flye
To see they torture us in vain
Sink idle in despair & dye

John Keats

(1795–1821)

Ode on Melancholy

No, no! go not to Lethe, neither twist
Wolf's-bane, tight-rooted, for its poisonous wine;
Nor suffer thy pale forehead to be kissed
By nightshade, ruby grape of Proserpine;
Make not your rosary of yew-berries,
Nor let the beetle nor the death-moth be
Your mournful Psyche, nor the downy owl
A partner in your sorrow's mysteries;
For shade to shade will come too drowsily,
And drown the wakeful anguish of the soul.

But when the melancholy fit shall fall
Sudden from heaven like a weeping cloud,
That fosters the droop-headed flowers all,
And hides the green hill in an April shroud;
Then glut thy sorrow on a morning rose,
Or on the rainbow of the salt sand-wave,
Or on the wealth of globed peonies;
Or if thy mistress some rich anger shows,
Emprison her soft hand, and let her rave,
And feed deep, deep upon her peerless eyes.

She dwells with Beauty—Beauty that must die;
And Joy, whose hand is ever at his lips
Bidding adieu; and aching Pleasure nigh,
Turning to poison while the bee-mouth sips;
Ay, in the very temple of delight
Veiled Melancholy has her sovran shrine,
Though seen of none save him whose strenuous tongue
Can burst Joy's grape against his palate fine;
His soul shall taste the sadness of her might,
And be among her cloudy trophies hung.

Anonymous ("Orestes")

(published 1796)

A Sonnet to Opium; Celebrating its Virtues. Written at the Side of Julia, when the Author was Inspired with a Dose of Laudanum, more than Sufficient for two moderate Turks

Soul-soothing drug! Your virtues let me laud,
   Which can with sov'reign sway
Force lawless passion into harmless play!
   Oft have I owned your pow'r
   In many a moody hour,
When grief with viper-tooth my heart hath gnawed.
   Still friendly to the plaintive muse,
   You can a balm infuse.
   If, sick with hopeless love,
   Too tenderly I mourn,
You can the shaft of anguish quick remove;
Or make desire's destructive flame less fiercely burn:
Guardian you are of Julia's innocence,
When madd'ning rapture goads to vice my throbbing sense.

Thomas Haynes Bayly

(1797–1839)

"I welcome thee back again, Spirit of Song!"

I welcome thee back again, Spirit of Song!
I've bent beneath sorrow's cold pressure too long.
I've suffered in silence; how vainly I sought
For words to unburthen the anguish of thought;
Despair haunts the silent endurance of wrong
I welcome thee back again, Spirit of Song!

I welcome thee back as the Dove to the Ark:
The world was a desert, the future all dark;
But I know that the worst of the storm must be past,
Thou art come with the green leaf of comfort at last.
Around me thy radiant imagining throng,
I welcome thee back again, Spirit of Song!

I feared thee, sweet Spirit! I thought thou would'st come
With memory's records of boyhood and home;
The home where I laughed away youth, and was told
It would still be my dwelling place when I grew old;
But visions of hope to thy coming belong,
I welcome thee back again, Spirit of Song!

Thou wilt not, sweet Spirit! thou wilt not, I know,
Mislead to the fruitless indulgence of woe,
That shrinks from the smile that would offer relief,
And seems to be proud of pre-eminent grief—
Thou'lt soothe the depression already too strong:
I welcome thee back again, Spirit of Song!

There's a chord that I never must venture to wake,
The sorrow a loved one hath borne for my sake;
But her love, which no change in my fortunes could chill,
Her smile of affection that follows me still,

Oh! these are the themes I may proudly prolong,
I welcome thee back again, Spirit of Song!

I welcome thee back, and again I look forth
With my wonted delight on the blessings of earth;
Again I can smile with the gay and the young;
The lamp is relighted, the harp is restrung.
Despair haunts the silent endurance of wrong,
I welcome thee back again, Spirit of Song!

Popular Songs: from *American Mock-Bird*

(published 1801)

The Mad Lover

What if I am mad? What if in pain
    I rave and rage and reel?
What if my tears, like scalding rain,
    Count every pang I feel.
Hadst thou fall'n victim to the art
    Of some false lovely she,
Heaven in her face, hell in her heart,
    Thou'd ave and rage like me.

I am Etna now, my bowels burn,
    Demons the lava blow;
And now I'm Caucasus and turn'd
    A chilling mass of snow.
Fool why dost laugh? where is the wit,
    With torture that makes free?
If hapless love thy brain had split,
    Thou'd freeze and burn like me.

On death's dread verge, I seem to stand,
    Yet hold my hated life:
To strike me down, no pitying hand,
    No poison cord or knife.
    Strike to my heart, ah, treacherous friend!
That will not set me free:
    Didst thou thus linger near thy end,
Thou'd long to die like me.

Crazy Paul

WHY, dear *George*, in every feature
    Are such signs of fear impress'd?
Can a mad, tho' hostile creature,
    With such terror fill thy breast?
Do his frenzied looks alarm thee?
    Let not these thy heart appal:
Not for *kingdoms can* he harm thee;. . . .
    Shun not then poor *Crazy Paul.*

Does *he* still for *Malta* languish?
    Mark him and avoid his woe;
Proud ambition causes anguish. . . .
    States are false. . . . *you* find them so.
Austria loves. . . . oh! how sincerely!
    While the guineas round her fall;
Denmark, Sweden, lov'd *as dearly,*
    Yet they're gone to *Crazy Paul.*

Fondly *George's* heart receiv'd *him,*
    Doom'd to court more kings than one;. . . .
Paul vow'd to love, and *George* believ'd him. . . .
    Paul is false. . . . *George not undone.*
From that hour his fleet is ready
    To attack with fire and ball;
Nelson with a courage steady,
    Cries, "*Have at thee, Crazy Paul.*"

British tars, so gallant-hearted,
    With victorious thoughts beset;
On seas where *they* and *Russia* parted,
    On seas where *they* and *Russia* met,
Still shall sing the war-lorn ditty,
    Still shall fight at *honor's* call;
While each passing *ship,* in pity,
    Cries, "*God help thee, Crazy Paul.*"

Popular Songs: from *Temple of Harmony*

(published 1801)

Song

LIFE'S as like as can be to an Irish wake,
    Where their tapers they light,
    And they sit up all night,
Wid their why would you leave your poor Paddy to moan,
Arrah how could you be such a cake?
    Musha what will I do?
    Lilly, lilly, lilly la loo,
    Oh hone!
    Fait we're left all together alone:
But when the grief the liquor puts out,
    The fun is all chang'o in a crack;
Away like smoke goes the whisky about,
    And they soot it, cross over, and back to back,
    With their tiptelery whack.

Poor miss, bolted safe with a good lock and key,
    Like Thisbe, may call
    Thro' the hole in the wall,
How hard's my misfortune, I'm left here to moan,
Will no one take pity on me?
    Musha, what will I do?
    Lilly, lilly, lilly la loo,
    Oh hone,
    I shall be after lying alone.
But when the rope-ladder affords her relief,
    And she turns on her mother her back;
Mong her friends and relations she leaves all her grief,
    And away to Scotland they trip in a crack,
    With their tiptelery whack.

The toper next morning, low, sick, and in pain,
    The glasses all breaks,
    Beats his head 'cause it aches,

151

And wishes that wine may a poison be grown,
    If e'er her gets tipsey again:
    With his what will I do,
    Lilly, lilly, lilly, la loo,
    Oh hone!
    From this moment I'll drinking disown;
But when in a possee, come Bacchus's troop,
    He changes his tone in a crack;
They drink and they sing, and they hollow and whoop,
    Till they don't know the color of blue from black,
And its tiptelary whack.

And so 'tis through life, widows left in the nick,
    Dying swains in disgrace,
    Patriots turn'd out of place,
Don't they, cursing their stars, make a horrible moan,
    Just like when the devil was sick?
    Wid their what will I do,
    Lilly, lilly, lilly, la loo,
    Oh hone!
    Fait we are left all to grunt and to groan;
But when the widow gets married again,
    When the lover is taken back,
When the patriot ousted a place shall obtain,
    Away to the devil goes care in a crack,
    And it's tiptelary whack.

Popular Songs: from *Choice Collection of Admired Songs*

(published 1805)

Crazy Jane

Why fair maid in every feature,
Are such signs of fear express'd;
Can a wandering wretched creature;
With such terror fill thy breast;
Do my frenzy'd looks alarm thee,
Trust me, sweet, thy fears are vain,
Not for kingdoms wou'd I harm thee,
Shun not then poor Crazy Jane.

Dost thou weep to feel my anguish?
Mark me, and avoid my woe;
When men flatter, sigh and languish,
Think them false, I found them so:
For I lov'd, Ah! so sincerely,
None could ever love again,
But the youth I lov'd so dearly,
Stole the wits of Crazy Jane.

Fondly my poor heart receiv'd him,
Which was doom'd to love but one,
He sigh'd, he vow'd and I believ'd him,
He was false and I undone;
From that hour has reason never
Held her empire o'er my brain;
Henry's fled, with him for ever,
Fled the wits of Crazy Jane.

Now forlorn and broken-hearted,
And with frenzied thoughts beset,
On that spot where last we parted,
On that spot where first we met:

Still I sing my love-lorn ditty,
Still I slowly pace the plain,
Whilst each passer-by in pity,
Cries God help thee Crazy Jane.

∽

The Death of Crazy Jane

'Twas at the hour, when night retreating,
Bade the screech-owl seek her nest;
Gloomy vapours flow were fleeting:
Morning glimmer'd in the East—
On the heath, her wild woes telling,
To the winds, and beating rain,
Cold, unshelter'd, far from dwelling,
Trembling fat poor Crazy Jane.

"Ah," she cried, "ye scenes around me,
Witnesses of Henry's art!
Witnesses he faithful found me—
How he broke this tender heart!
Go ye wild winds! try to move him,
Bid him heal this heart again!—
Did he know how much I love him,
He would pity Crazy Jane!

"Henry comes! I see him yonder,
Dart like ligh'ning o'er the heath,
Ah, no! no!—my senses wander!
Since he comes not, welcome Death!"
Fainting, on the heath she laid her;
Soon, in pity to her pain,
Death, where Love at first betray'd her;
Gave relief to Crazy Jane.

Popular Songs: from *Boston Musical Miscellany*

(published 1815)

Nancy and Gin

From a flasket of gin, my dear Nancy requested
A glass her sweet spirits to cheer;
"No, by heav'ns!" I exclaim'd, "may I perish
If ever I give such sad trash to my dear."

When I shew'd her the ring, and implor'd her to marry,
She frown'd like a dark foggy morn;
"No, by heav'ns!" she exclaim'd, "may I perish
For such a sad niggard sure never was born."

I press'd her dear fist, but she look'd like a fury,
And snatch'd it away full of scorn,
"No, by heav'n!" she exclaim'd, "I'll ne'er marry
Unless that a dram I may have night and morn."

Popular Songs: from *Songster's Companion*

(published 1815)

Mary Le More

As I stray'd o'er a common on Cork's rugged border,
    While the dew-drops of morn the sweet primrose array'd,
I saw a poor female, whose mental disorder,
    Her quick glancing eye wild aspect betray'd;
On the sward she reclin'd, by the green fern surrounded,
At her side speckled daises and crow flowers abounded;
To its inmost recess her poor heart had been wounded;
    Her sighs were unceasing, 'twas Mary Le More.

Her charms by the keen blast of sorrow were faded,
    Yet the soft tinge of beauty still play'd on her cheek;
Her tresses a wreath of pale primroses braided,
    And strings of fresh daises hung loose on her neck;
While with pity I gaz'd, she exclaim'd, "O! my mother!
See the blood on that lash, 'tis the blood of my brother;
They have torn his poor flesh, and they now strip another;
    'Tis Connor, the friend of poor Mary Le More!"

"Though his locks are as white as the foam of the ocean,
    Those soldiers shall find that my father is brave;
My father!" she cry'd, with the wildest emotion,
    "Ah! no, my poor father now sleeps in the grave!
They have toll'd his death bell, they've laid the turf o'er him;
His white locks were bloody, no aid can restore him;
He is gone! he is gone! the good will deplore him,
    When the blue wave of Erin hides Mary Le More!"

A lark, from the gold blossom'd furze that grew near her,
    Now rose, and with energy caroll'd his lay;
"Hush! hush! she continued, the trumpet sounds clearer;
    The horsemen approach: Erin's daughters away!
Ah! Britons, 'twas foul, while the cabin was burning,
And o'er her pale father a wretch had been mourning!

Go hide with the sea mew, ye maids, and take warning;
　　Those ruffians have ruin'd poor Mary Le More."

"Away! bring the ointment! O God! see those gashes,
　　Alas! my poor mother, come dry the big tear;
Anon we'll have vengeance for those dreadful lashes
　　Already the screech-owl and ravens appear;
By day the green grave, that lies under the willow,
With wild flowers I'll strew, and by night make my pillow;
Till the ooze and dark sea weed, beneath the curl'd billow,
　　Shall furnish a death bed for Mary Le More."

Thus rav'd the poor Maniac in tones more heart-rending
　　Than sanity's voice ever pour'd on my ear,
When, lo! on the waste, and their march t'ward her bending
　　A troop of fierce cavalry chanc'd to appear
"Oh! fiends!" she exclaim'd, and with wild horror started,
Then thro' the tall fern, loudly screaming, she darted;
With an overcharg'd bosom, I slowly departed,
And sigh'd for the wrongs of poor Mary Le More.

Away with Melancholy

AWAY with melancholy,
Nor doleful changes ring,
On life and human folly,
But merrily merrily sing, fal la.

Come on ye rosy hours,
Gay smiling moments bring;
We'll strew the way with flow'rs
And merrily merrily sing, fal la.

For what's the use of sighing
Since time is on the wing,
Can we prevent its flying?
Then merrily merrily sing fal la.

Popular Songs: from *Songs for Ladies*

(published 1825)

The Frantic Maid

To Mary's sad story, give ear gentle stranger,
   And pity those woes which we cannot remove;
A poor frantic maid! o'er the wide earth a ranger,
   She talks to the moon, and she asks for her love.

She once was as fair as the white blooming thorn,
   While yet on its blossom the dew drop is hung;
She once was as gay as the bright summer's morn,
   And down by yon cottage she cheerfully sung.

But now the poor maniac sits by the willow,
   All the long night by the rivulet's side;
And here Henry, she says, lies low in the billow,
   For bravely he fought, and in battle he died.

Poor Mary, she wanders with uncover'd feet,
   And gathers a garland to hand on each spray;
And sings a sad ditty, more plaintively sweet,
   Than the Wood-lark's wild note at the close of the day.

Popular Songs: from *The Muse, or The Flowers of Poetry*

(published 1827)

Soliloquy on Smoking

To smoke—or not to smoke—that is the question
Whether 'tis better to abjure the habit,
And trust the warnings of a scribbling doctor,
Or buy at once a box of best Havana,
And, ten a day, consume them? To smoke—to puff—
Nay, more, to waste the tender fabric of the lungs,
And risk consumption, and the thousand ills
The practice leads to; 'tis a consummation
Discreetly to be shunn'd. To smoke—to puff—
To puff—perchance to doze—ay, there's the rub;
For in that dozing state we thirsty grow;
And, having burnt the tube up to a stump,
We must have drink—and that's one cause
We modern youth are destin'd to short life.
For who can bear to feel his mouth parch'd up,
His throat like whalebone, and his chest exhausted,
His head turn giddy, and his nerves unstrung,
When he himself might drench these ills away
With wine or brandy? Who would live in smoke,
And pine and sicken with a secret poison,
But the dread of breaking o'er a rule,
Prescrib'd by fashion, (whose controlling will
None disobeys,) puzzles ambitious youth,
And makes us rather bear those ills we feel,
And others, that the doctor warns us of?
Thus custom does make spectres of us all;
And thus the native hue of our complexion
As sicklied o'er with pale, consumptive cast;
The appetite, (a loss of greater moment,)
Pall'd by the weed, and the digestive pow'rs
Lose all their action.

Elizabeth Barrett Browning

(1806–1861)

Grief

I tell you, hopeless grief is passionless
That only men incredulous of despair,
Half-taught in anguish, through the midnight air
Beat upward to God's throne in loud access
Of shrieking and reproach. Full desertness,
In souls as countries, lieth silent-bare
Under the blanching, vertical eye-glare
Of the absolute Heavens. Deep-hearted man, express
Grief for thy Dead in silence like to death—
Most like a monumental statue set
In everlasting watch and moveless woe
Till itself crumble to the dust beneath.
Touch it; the marble eyelids are not wet:
If it could weep, it could arise and go.

Alfred Tennyson

(1809–1892)

from **"In Memoriam"**

. . .

III

O Sorrow, cruel fellowship,
   O Priestess in the vaults of Death,
   O sweet and bitter in a breath,
What whispers from thy lying lip?

"The stars," she whispers, "blindly run;
   A web is wov'n across the sky;
   From out waste places comes a cry,
And murmurs from the dying sun:

"And all the phantom, Nature, stands—
   With all the music in her tone,
   A hollow echo of my own,—
A hollow form with empty hands."

And shall I take a thing so blind,
   Embrace her as my natural good;
   Or crush her, like a vice of blood,
Upon the threshold of the mind?

IV

To Sleep I give my powers away;
   My will is bondsman to the dark;
   I sit within a helmless bark,
And with my heart I muse and say:

O heart, how fares it with thee now,
   That thou should'st fail from thy desire,
   Who scarcely darest to inquire,
"What is it makes me beat so low?"

Something it is which thou hast lost,
 Some pleasure from thine early years.
 Break, thou deep vase of chilling tears,
That grief hath shaken into frost!

Such clouds of nameless trouble cross
 All night below the darken'd eyes;
 With morning wakes the will, and cries,
"Thou shalt not be the fool of loss."

  V
I sometimes hold it half a sin
 To put in words the grief I feel;
 For words, like Nature, half reveal
And half conceal the Soul within

But, for the unquiet heart and brain,
 A use in measured language lies;
 The sad mechanic exercise,
Like dull narcotics, numbing pain.

In words, like weeds, I'll wrap me o'er,
 Like coarsest clothes against the cold:
 But that large grief which these enfold
Is given in outline and no more.

   . . .

  XVI
What words are these have fall'n from me?
 Can calm despair and wild unrest
 Be tenants of a single breast,
Or sorrow such a changeling be?

Or doth she only seem to take
 The touch of change in calm or storm;
 But knows no more of transient form
In her deep self, than some dead lake

That holds the shadow of a lark
 Hung in the shadow of a heaven?

Or has the shock, so harshly given,
Confused me like the unhappy bark

That strikes by night a craggy shelf,
    And staggers blindly ere she sink?
    And stunn'd me from my power to think
And all my knowledge of myself;

And made me that delirious man
    Whose fancy fuses old and new,
    And flashes into false and true,
And mingles all without a plan?

                . . .

    XIX
The Danube to the Severn gave
    The darken'd heart that beat no more;
    They laid him by the pleasant shore,
And in the hearing of the wave.

There twice a day the Severn fills;
    The salt sea-water passes by,
    And hushes half the babbling Wye,
And makes a silence in the hills.

The Wye is hush'd nor moved along,
    And hush'd my deepest grief of all,
    When fill'd with tears that cannot fall,
I brim with sorrow drowning song.

The tide flows down, the wave again
    Is vocal in its wooded walls;
    My deeper anguish also falls,
And I can speak a little then.

                . . .

Matthew Arnold

(1822–1888)

from "Empedocles on Etna"

Callicles:
But oh! Pausanias, he is changed of late;
There is a settled trouble in his air
Admits no momentary brightening now,
And when he comes among his friends at feasts,
'Tis as an orphan among prosperous boys.
Thou know'st of old he loved this harp of mine,
When first he sojourned with Peisianax;
He is now always moody, and I fear him;
But I would serve him, soothe him, if I could,
Dared one but try.

. . .

Empedocles:
And lie thou there,
My laurel bough!
Scornful Apollo's ensign, lie thou there!
Though thou hast been my shade in the world's heat,
Though I have loved thee, lived in honoring thee,
Yet lie thou there,
My laurel bough!

I am weary of thee.
I am weary of the solitude
Where he who bears thee must abide,—
Of the rocks of Parnassus,
Of the gorge of Delphi,
Of the moonlit peaks, and the caves.
Thou guardest them, Apollo!
Over the grave of the slain Pytho,
Though young, intolerably severe!
Thou keepest aloof the profane,

But the solitude oppresses thy votary!
The jars of men reach him not in thy valley,

But can life reach him?
Thou fencest him from the multitude:
Who will fence him from himself?
He hears nothing but the cry of the torrents,
And the beating of his own heart;
The air is thin, the veins swell,
The temples tighten and throb there—
Air! air!

Take thy bough, set me free from my solitude;
I have been enough alone!

Where shall thy votary fly then? back to men?
But they will gladly welcome him once more,
And help him to unbend his too tense thought,
And rid him of the presence of himself,
And keep their friendly chatter at his ear,
And haunt him, till the absence from himself,
That other torment, grow unbearable;
And he will fly to solitude again,
And he will find its air too keen for him,
And so change back; and many thousand times
Be miserably bandied to and fro
Like a sea-wave, betwixt the world and thee,
Thou young, implacable God! and only death
Can cut his oscillations short, and so
Bring him to poise. There is no other way.

. . .

And thou, fiery world,
That sapp'st the vitals of this terrible mount
Upon whose charred and quaking crust I stand—
Thou, too, brimmest with life!—the sea of cloud,
That heaves its white and billowy vapors up
To moat this isle of ashes from the world,
Lives; and that other fainter sea, far down,
O'er whose lit floor a road of moonbeams leads
To Etna's Liparëan sister-fires
And the long dusky line of Italy—

165

That mild and luminous floor of waters lives,
With held-in joy swelling its heart; I only,
Whose spring of hope is dried, whose spirit has failed,
I, who have not, like these, in solitude
Maintained courage and force, and in myself
Nursed an immortal vigor—I alone
Am dead to life and joy, therefore I read
In all things my own deadness.

A long silence. He continues:—

Oh, that I could glow like this mountain!
Oh, that my heart bounded with the swell of the sea!
Oh, that my soul were full of light as the stars!
Oh, that it brooded over the world like the air!

But no, this heart will glow no more; thou art
A living man no more, Empedocles!
Nothing but a devouring flame of thought—
But a naked, eternally restless mind!

. . .

        Slave of sense
I have in no wise been;—but slave of thought?
And who can say: I have been always free,
Lived ever in the light of my own soul?
I cannot; I have lived in wrath and gloom,
Fierce, disputatious, ever at war with man,
Far from my own soul, far from warmth and light;
But I have not grown easy in these bonds,
But I have not denied what bonds these were.
Yea, I take myself to witness,
That I have loved no darkness,
Sophisticated no truth,
Nursed no delusion,
Allowed no fear!

And therefore, O ye elements! I know—
Ye know it too—it hath been granted me
Not to die wholly, not to be all enslaved.
I feel it in this hour. The numbing cloud
Mounts off my soul; I feel it, I breathe free.

Is it but for a moment?
—Ah, boil up, ye vapors!
Leap and roar, thou sea of fire!
My soul glows to meet you.
Ere it flag, ere the mists
Of despondency and gloom
Rush over it again,
Receive me, save me!

He plunges into the crater.

Sydney Dobell

(1824–1874)

from "Balder. Part The First," Scenes XIII & XIV

. . .

Happier to drive
The patient ass along the beaten way,
Laden with humble fruits to the set mart
Of fixed reward, and back to certain rest,
And sweet assured possession, than like me
Bound helpless on the fury of the winds,
To scour the plains I seek not, scale the height
Where my brain swims, and leap, as in a dream,
Down into the unfathomable void,
While from the fall—like my back-streaming hair—
Fear-blown in all my veins the blood streams back,
And faints with horror.

I that am called proud,
Lying most humbly weary and abject
On the immoveable earth that doth so please
This mortal frame, and seeing my dull race
Doing their easy pleasures to and fro,
Self-ordinate, could sometimes sell my birth-right
For any pottage that would feed the flesh
Of other men upon me.

Death, Death, Death!
I have seen every face but thine to-day!
And to behold thee, from sunrise till now, How have I strained
    these eyeballs

. . .

The fourth time the strong silence in the cell
Was as the straining silence of the rack,
When the still-tightening torture wrenches him
Who will not speak. The great veins in my brow

Throbbed with suppression, and such consciousness
I had of coming uproar, rising up
Thro' the containing stillness—as the fire
Of Ætna swells under her dark blind hill
And bursts in desolation—that my lips
Cried out. As if the sudden whip of Hell
Flashed on a pack of demons caught asleep,
The place brake silence, and a naked shriek
Came thro' the right-hand wall and, shrieking, passed
Out on the left, and when I called, returned,
Still shrieking, and so out upon the right,
And to and fro until my deafened brain
Reeled, and I fell down flat and slept as dead.
Then to me, sleeping, in my ear, these words,
Not as from outer nature, yet in voice
Not mine, tho' nearer to me than the ear
That heard it, as if in my head the blood
Along the intricate deep veins did hiss
A whisper and fled shivering to the heart.
'Bring me the inflated skin thou callest Life,
And I will turn the wind-bag inside out
And clothe me.'

              I am not the fool of dreams,
Yet hold it not incredible that things
Are seen before their time, and,—as to-night
In this strange vision, where, while all was still
I felt the undelivered silence swell—
Somewhat to be lies in the womb of Now,
And eyes unstayed by mortal obscuration
Behold at once the Mother and the Child.
A white skin and the sweet fair-seeming flesh
Shut back the common eye-sight; but there be
Who looking fast on the unblushed repose
Of Beauty—where she lieth bright and still
As some spent angel, dead-asleep in light
On the most heavenward top of all this world,
Wing-weary—seized with sudden trance and strong
Thro' the decorous continent and all
The charmed defence of Nature can behold
The circling health beneath them, the red haste
Of the quick heart, and of her heaving breast

169

The cavernous and windy mysteries;
Yea, all the creeping secrets of her maw,
The busy rot within her, and the worm
That preys upon her vitals. So perchance
I see the Future in the Present. Or
If in the smoothest hour of patent nature
That overhanging weight of Destiny
Which loads the heavy air do brood on us,
What wonder that our tenderer substance take
Impress divine, and show the awful stamp
And parody of Fate?

          One can be brave
At noon, and with triumphant logic clear
The demonstrable air, but ne'ertheless,
Sometimes at Hallowe'en when, legends say,
The things that stir among the rustling trees
Are not all mortal, and the sick white moon
Wanes o'er the season of the sheeted dead,
We grow unreasonable and do quake
With more than the cold wind. The very soul,
Sick as the moon, suspects her sentinels,
And thro' her fortress of the body peers
Shivering abroad; our heart-strings over-strung,
Scare us with strange involuntary notes
Quivering and quaking, and the creeping flesh
Knows all the starting horrors of surprise
But that which makes them, and for that, half-wild,
Quickens the winking lids, and glances out
From side to side, as if some sudden chance
Of vision, some unused slant of the eye,
Some accidental focus of the sight
O' th' instant might reveal a peopled world
Crowding about us, and the empty light
Alive with phantoms. Doubtless there are no ghosts;
Yet somehow it is better not to move
Lest cold hands seize upon us from behind,
Or forward thro' the dim uncertain time
Face close with paly face. My ominous Dream
Leaves me in shuddering incredulity
As logically white.

            · · ·

Emily Dickinson

(1830–1886)

#126

To fight aloud, is very brave—
But *gallanter*, I know
Who charge within the bosom
The Cavalry of Woe—

Who win, and nations do not see—
Who fall—and none observe—
Whose dying eyes, no Country
Regards with patriot love—

We trust, in plumed procession
For such, the Angels go—
Rank after Rank, with even feet—
And Uniforms of Snow.

#410

The first Day's Night had come—
And grateful that a thing
So terrible—had been endured—
I told my Soul to sing—

She said her Strings were snapt—
Her Bow—to Atoms blown—
And so to mend her—gave me work
Until another Morn—

And then—a Day as huge
As Yesterdays in pairs,
Unrolled its horror in my face—
Until it blocked my eyes—

My Brain—begun to laugh—
I mumbled—like a fool—
And tho' 'tis Years ago—that Day—
My Brain keeps giggling—still.

And Something's odd—within—
That person that I was—
And this One—do not feel the same—
Could it be Madness—this?

#435

Much Madness is divinest Sense—
To a discerning Eye—
Much Sense—the starkest Madness—
'Tis the Majority
In this, as All, prevail—
Assent—and you are sane—
Demur—you're straightway dangerous—
And handled with a Chain—

#670

One need not be a Chamber—to be Haunted—
One need not be a House—

The Brain has Corridors—surpassing
Material Place—

Far safer, of a Midnight Meeting
External Ghost
Than its interior Confronting—
That Cooler Host.

Far safer, through an Abbey gallop,
The Stones a'chase—
Than Unarmed, one's a'self encounter—
In lonesome Place—

Ourself behind ourself, concealed—
Should startle most—
Assassin hid in our Apartment
Be Horror's least.

The Body—borrows a Revolver—
He bolts the Door—
O'erlooking a superior spectre—
Or More—

#1062

He scanned it—staggered—
Dropped the Loop
To Past or Period—
Caught helpless at a sense as if
His Mind were going blind—

Groped up, to see if God was there—
Groped backward at Himself
Caressed a Trigger absently
And wandered out of Life.

Henry Kendall

(1839–1882)

Outre Mer

I see, as one in dreaming,
  A broad, bright, quiet sea;
Beyond it lies a haven—
  The only home for me.
Some men grow strong with trouble,
  But all my strength is past,
And tired and full of sorrow
  I long to sleep at last.
By force of chance and changes
  Man's life is hard at best;
And, seeing rest is voiceless,
  The dearest thing is rest.

Beyond the sea—behold it,
  The home I wish to seek,
The refuge of the weary,
  The solace of the weak!
Sweet angel fingers beckon,
  Sweet angel voices ask
My soul to cross the waters;
  And yet I dread the task.
God help the man whose trials
  Are tares that he must reap;
He cannot face the future—
  His only hope is sleep.

Across the main a vision
  Of sunset coasts, and skies,
And widths of waters gleaming,
  Enchant my human eyes.
I, who have sinned and suffered,
  Have sought—with tears have sought—

To rule my life with goodness,
 And shape it to my thought.
And yet there is no refuge
 To shield me from distress,
Except the realm of slumber
 And great forgetfulness.

Thomas Hardy

(1840–1928)

Just the Same

I sat. It all was past;
Hope never would hail again;
Fair days had ceased at a blast,
The world was a darkened den.

The beauty and dream were gone,
And the halo in which I had hied
So gaily gallantly on
Had suffered blot and died!

I went forth, heedless whither,
In a cloud too black for name:
—People frisked hither and thither;
The world was just the same.

The Wound

I climbed to the crest,
    And, fog-festooned,
The sun lay west
    Like a crimson wound:

Like that wound of mine
    Of which none knew,
For I'd given no sign
    That it pierced me through.

In Tenebris II

When the clouds' swoln bosoms echo back the shouts of the many
    and strong
That things are all as they best may be, save a few to be right ere long,
And my eyes have not the vision in them to discern what to these is
    so clear,
The blot seems straightway in me alone; one better he were not here.

The stout upstanders say, All's well with us: ruers have nought to rue!
And what the potent say so oft, can it fail to be somewhat true?
Breezily go they, breezily come; their dust smokes around their career,
Till I think I am one born out of due time, who has no calling here.

Their dawns bring lusty joys, it seems; their evenings all that is sweet;
Our times are blessed times, they cry: Life shapes it as is most meet,
And nothing is much the matter; there are many smiles to a tear;
Then what is the matter is I, I say. Why should such an one be here? . . .

Let him in whose ears the low-voiced Best is killed by the clash
    of the First,
Who holds that if way to the Better there be, it exacts a full look
    at the Worst,
Who feels that delight is a delicate growth cramped by crookedness,
    custom, and fear,
Get him up and be gone as one shaped awry; he disturbs the
    order here.

Mad Judy

When the hamlet hailed a birth
    Judy used to cry:
When she heard our christening mirth
    She would kneel and sigh.
She was crazed, we knew, and we
Humoured her infirmity.

When the daughters and the sons
   Gathered them to wed,
And we like-intending ones
   Danced till dawn was red,
She would rock and mutter, "More
Comers to this stony shore!"

When old Headsman Death laid hands
   On a babe or twain,
She would feast, and by her brands
   Sing her songs again.
What she liked we let her do,
Judy was insane, we knew.

Robert Bridges

(1844–1930)

Melancholia

The sickness of desire, that in dark days
Looks on the imagination of despair,
Forgetteth man, and stinteth God his praise;
Nor but in sleep findeth a cure for care.
Incertainty that once gave scope to dream
Of laughing enterprise and glory untold,
Is now a blackness that no stars redeem,
A wall of terror in a night of cold.
Fool! thou that hast impossibly desired
And now impatiently despairest, see
How nought is changed: Joy's wisdom is attired
Splendid for others' eyes if not for thee:
Not love or beauty or youth from earth is fled:
If they delite thee not, 'tis thou art dead.

Gerard Manley Hopkins

(1844–1889)

"No worst, there is none. Pitched past pitch of grief"

No worst, there is none. Pitched past pitch of grief,
More pangs will, schooled at forepangs, wilder wring.
Comforter, where, where is your comforting?
Mary, mother of us, where is your relief?
My cries heave, herds-long; huddle in a main, a chief
Woe, world-sorrow; on an age-old anvil wince and sing—
Then lull, then leave off. Fury had shrieked 'No ling-
ering! Let me be fell: force I must be brief.'

O the mind, mind has mountains; cliffs of fall
Frightful, sheer, no-man-fathomed. Hold them cheap
May who ne'er hung there. Nor does long our small
Durance deal with that steep or deep. Here! creep,
Wretch, under a comfort serves in a whirlwind: all
Life death does end and each day dies with sleep.

Carrion Comfort

Not, I'll not, carrion comfort, Despair, not feast on thee;
Not untwist—slack they may be—these last strands of man
In me ór, most weary, cry *I can no more*. I can;
Can something, hope, wish day come, not choose not to be.
But ah, but O thou terrible, why wouldst thou rude on me
Thy wring-world right foot rock? lay a lionlimb against me? scan
With darksome devouring eyes my bruisèd bones? and fan,
O in turns of tempest, me heaped there; me frantic to avoid thee
    and flee?

Why? That my chaff might fly; my grain lie, sheer and clear.
Nay in all that toil, that coil, since (seems) I kissed the rod,
Hand rather, my heart lo! lapped strength, stole joy, would laugh,
    chéer.
Cheer whom though? the hero whose heaven-handling flung me,
    fóot tród
Me? or me that fought him? O which one? is it each one? That night,
    that year
Of now done darkness I wretch lay wrestling with (my God!) my God.

"I wake and feel the fell of dark, not day"

I wake and feel the fell of dark, not day.
What hours, O what black hours we have spent
This night! what sights you, heart, saw; ways you went!
And more must, in yet longer light's delay.

With witness I speak this. But where I say
Hours I mean years, mean life. And my lament
Is cries countless, cries like dead letters sent
To dearest him that lives alas! away.

I am gall, I am heartburn. God's most deep decrees
Bitter would have me taste: my taste was me;
Bones built in me, flesh filled, blood brimmed the curse.

Selfyeast of spirit a dull dough sours. I see
The lost are like this, and their scourge to be
As I am mine, their sweating selves, but worse.

A. Mary F. Robinson

(1857–1944)

Neurasthenia

I watch the happier people of the house
   Come in and out, and talk, and go their ways;
I sit and gaze at them; I cannot rouse
   My heavy mind to share their busy days.

I watch them glide, like skaters on a stream,
   Across the brilliant surface of the world.
But I am underneath: they do not dream
   How deep below the eddying flood is whirl'd.

They cannot come to me, nor I to them;
   But, if a mightier arm could reach and save,
Should I forget the tide I had to stem?
   Should I, like these, ignore the abysmal wave?

Yes! in the radiant air how could I know
How black it is, how fast it is, below?

Ernest Dowson

(1867–1900)

To One in Bedlam

With delicate, mad hands, behind his sordid bars,
Surely he hath his posies, which they tear and twine;
Those scentless wisps of straw, that miserably line
His strait, caged universe, whereat the dull world stares,

Pedant and pitiful. O, how his rapt gaze wars
With their stupidity! Know they what dreams divine
Lift his long, laughing reveries like enchanted wine,
And make his melancholy germane to the stars?

O lamentable brother! if those pity thee,
Am I not fain of all thy lone eyes promise me;
Half a fool's kingdom, far from men who sow and reap,
All their days, vanity? Better than mortal flowers,
Thy moon-kissed roses seem: better than love or sleep,
The star-crowned solitude of thine oblivious hours!

Spleen

I was not sorrowful, I could not weep,
And all my memories were put to sleep.

I watched the river grow more white and strange,
All day till evening I watched it change.

All day till evening I watched the rain
Beat wearily upon the window pane

I was not sorrowful, but only tired
Of everything that ever I desired.

Her lips, her eyes, all day became to me
The shadow of a shadow utterly.

All day mine hunger for her heart became
Oblivion, until the evening came,

And left me sorrowful, inclined to weep,
With all my memories that could not sleep.

Edward Thomas

(1878–1917)

Melancholy

The rain and wind, the rain and wind, raved endlessly.
On me the Summer storm, and fever, and melancholy
Wrought magic, so that if I feared the solitude
Far more I feared all company: too sharp, too rude,
Had been the wisest or the dearest human voice.
What I desired I knew not, but whate'er my choice
Vain it must be, I knew. Yet naught did my despair
But sweeten the strange sweetness, while through the wild air
All day long I heard a distant cuckoo calling
And, soft as dulcimers, sounds of near water falling,
And, softer, and remote as if in history,
Rumours of what had touched my friends, my foes, or me.

Rain

Rain, midnight rain, nothing but the wild rain
On this bleak hut, and solitude, and me
Remembering again that I shall die
And neither hear the rain nor give it thanks
For washing me cleaner than I have been
Since I was born into this solitude.
Blessed are the dead that the rain rains upon:
But here I pray that none whom once I loved
Is dying to-night or lying still awake
Solitary, listening to the rain,

Either in pain or thus in sympathy
Helpless among the living and the dead,
Like a cold water among broken reeds,
Myriads of broken reeds all still and stiff,
Like me who have no love which this wild rain
Has not dissolved except the love of death,
If love it be for what is perfect and
Cannot, the tempest tells me, disappoint.

Siegfried Sassoon

(1886–1967)

Repression of War Experience

Now light the candles; one; two; there's a moth;
What silly beggars they are to blunder in
And scorch their wings with glory, liquid flame—
No, no, not that,—it's bad to think of war,
When thoughts you've gagged all day come back to scare you;
And it's been proved that soldiers don't go mad
Unless they lose control of ugly thoughts
That drive them out to jabber among the trees.

Now light your pipe; look, what a steady hand.
Draw a deep breath; stop thinking; count fifteen,
And you're as right as rain . . .
Why won't it rain? . . .
I wish there'd be a thunder-storm to-night,
With bucketsful of water to sluice the dark,
And make the roses hang their dripping heads.
Books; what a jolly company they are,
Standing so quiet and patient on their shelves,
Dressed in dim brown, and black, and white, and green,
And every kind of colour. Which will you read?
Come on; O do read something; they're so wise.
I tell you all the wisdom of the world
Is waiting for you on those shelves; and yet
You sit and gnaw your nails, and let your pipe out,
And listen to the silence: on the ceiling
There's one big, dizzy moth that bumps and flutters;
And in the breathless air outside the house
The garden waits for something that delays.
There must be crowds of ghosts among the trees,—
Not people killed in battle,—they're in France,—
But horrible shapes in shrouds—old men who died
Slow, natural deaths,—old men with ugly souls,
Who wore their bodies out with nasty sins.

You're quiet and peaceful, summering safe at home;
You'd never think there was a bloody war on! . . .
O yes, you would . . . why, you can hear the guns.
Hark! Thud, thud, thud,—quite soft . . . they never cease—
Those whispering guns—O Christ, I want to go out
And screech at them to stop—I'm going crazy;
I'm going stark, staring mad because of the guns.

Haunted

Evening was in the wood, louring with storm.
A time of drought had sucked the weedy pool
And baked the channels; birds had done with song.
Thirst was a dream of fountains in the moon,
Or willow-music blown across the water
Leisurely sliding on by weir and mill.

Uneasy was the man who wandered, brooding,
His face a little whiter than the dusk.
A drone of sultry wings flicker'd in his head.
The end of sunset burning thro' the boughs
Died in a smear of red; exhausted hours
Cumber'd, and ugly sorrows hemmed him in.

He thought: 'Somewhere there's thunder,' as he strove
To shake off dread; he dared not look behind him,
But stood, the sweat of horror on his face.
He blunder'd down a path, trampling on thistles,
In sudden race to leave the ghostly trees.
And: 'Soon I'll be in open fields,' he thought,
And half remembered starlight on the meadows,
Scent of mown grass and voices of tired men,
Fading along the field-paths; home and sleep
And cool-swept upland spaces, whispering leaves,
And far off the long churring night-jar's note.

But something in the wood, trying to daunt him,
Led him confused in circles through the thicket.
He was forgetting his old wretched folly,
And freedom was his need; his throat was choking.
Barbed brambles gripped and clawed him round his legs,
And he floundered over snags and hidden stumps.
Mumbling: 'I will get out! I must get out!'
Butting and thrusting up the baffling gloom,
Pausing to listen in a space 'twixt thorns,
He peers around with peering, frantic eyes.
An evil creature in the twilight looping,
Flapped blindly in his face. Beating it off,
He screeched in terror, and straightway something clambered
Heavily from an oak, and dropped, bent double,
To shamble at him zigzag, squat and bestial.
Headlong he charges down the wood, and falls
With roaring brain—agony—the snap't spark—
And blots of green and purple in his eyes.
Then the slow fingers groping on his neck,
And at his heart the strangling clasp of death.

Ivor Gurney

(1890–1937)

Strange Hells

There are strange hells within the minds war made
Not so often, not so humiliatingly afraid
As one would have expected—the racket and fear guns made.
One hell the Gloucester soldiers they quite put out:
Their first bombardment, when in combined black shout

Of fury, guns aligned, they ducked lower their heads
And sang with diaphragms fixed beyond all dreads,
That tin and stretched-wire tinkle, that blither of tune:
'Après la guerre fini,' till hell all had come down,
Twelve-inch, six-inch, and eighteen pounders hammering
    hell's thunders.

Where are they now, on state-doles, or showing shop-patterns
Or walking town to town sore in borrowed tatterns
Or begged. Some civic routine one never learns.
The heart burns—but has to keep out of face how heart burns.

The Shame

If the pain I suffer were of the Devil enemy of man
It might pass, might be proper, but from man's self, O the
    black shame
Of torture, when, as some think, so easy were the plan
Of kind life; but this is dreadfulness beyond name.

Each minute packed with a badness beyond words,
The brain, the mind tortured as blind stones would do,
What help in life? None. Hope is that death affords
A shelter in some shade beyond pain's come-through.

What help? Who tortures? and why? Why not grant death
Which ends all, as some hope, and that Romans would think
An expiation complete: offence ended with breath.
And self killing as good a deed as ever were drink.

To God

Why have you made life so intolerable
And set me between four walls, where I am able
Not to escape meals without prayer, for that is possible
Only by annoying an attendant. And tonight a sensual
Hell has been put on me, so that all has deserted me
And I am merely crying and trembling in heart
For death, and cannot get it. And gone out is part
Of sanity. And there is dreadful hell within me.
And nothing helps. Forced meals there have been and electricity
And weakening of sanity by influence
That's dreadful to endure. And there is Orders
And I am praying for death, death, death,
And dreadful is the indrawing or out-breathing of breath
Because of the intolerable insults put on my whole soul,
Of the soul loathed, loathed, loathed of the soul.
Gone out every bright thing from my mind.
All lost that ever God himself designed.
Not half can be written of cruelty of man, on man,
Not often such evil guessed as between man and man.

An Appeal for Death

There is one who all day wishes to die,
And appeals for it—without a reason why—
Since Death is easy if men are merciful.
Water and land with chances are packed full.
Who all day wishes to die. How many ages
Have denied Death so—who reads old-written pages
And finds 'This man suffered and prayed for Death,
And went beyond this, desire of life beneath'?
Bitterly, bitterly, and though he feels his wrongs,
And once took pride in verse-making and in songs,
Yet now, yet now would wish to rest, and be
Out of pain, out of life, quietly, as quietly
As pained men ever were meant to rest.
Humanity knows earth to have as quiet a breast
As ever mother's to a longing child.
Therefore in mercy let rest, let rest this wild,
Or show hard torment, or of fear of such
Let rest, out of the fear of any pain's touch.
If men will not honour, nor find employ,
Will common mercy not forget what was wrong,
Remember what was good—a maker of song
Asks, desires, has prayed for mercy of Death
To end all, lie still, quiet green turf beneath,
Since promises forgotten are, and friendliness
Between so many men and him? The address
Of courtesy to casual wayfarers,
Small presents, courtesy of peace and wars—
To rest from pain, to trouble no one more—
Under green turf-mound, or by friendly shore
That will with rocking water lull his peace
That cannot now find hope nor strength nor ease.
To be let rest in mercy—to know an end
Of surety, Death's quiet surest of friend,
And what men would not, let calm Nature mend.

For Mercy of Death

I suffer racking pain all day, and desire death so—
As few desire. Where is man's mercy gone?
Did ever past generations such torment know
Who lived near earth, and joyed when the sun shone,
Or when sweet rain came on
The earth; and the afterglow
Of sun and flowers in show
Of golden sweetness gladdened earth's dear son?
Where is that mercy now
That palpably took pleasure in the sweep
Of hedgerows—high to deep—
And houses in the making, man's own dear
Vesture and shelter here?
O sure it is that if those olden-time
Builders of farm and byre
Were here again, my pain should pity receive—
Death should make no more to grieve
My spirit with such pain it knows not how
To endure. O show
Such olden pity on poor souls in pain.
Let rest again—
As would our fathers, friends of wind and rain.

Wilfred Owen

(1893–1918)

Mental Cases

Who are these? Why sit they here in twilight?
Wherefore rock they, purgatorial shadows,
Drooping tongues from jays that slob their relish,
Baring teeth that leer like skulls' teeth wicked?
Stroke on stroke of pain,—but what slow panic,
Gouged these chasms round their fretted sockets?
Ever from their hair and through their hands' palms
Misery swelters. Surely we have perished
Sleeping, and walk hell; but who these hellish?

—These are men whose minds the Dead have ravished.
Memory fingers in their hair of murders,
Multitudinous murders they once witnessed.
Wading sloughs of flesh these helpless wander,
Treading blood from lungs that had loved laughter.
Always they must see these things and hear them,
Batter of guns and shatter of flying muscles,
Carnage incomparable, and human squander
Rucked too thick for these men's extrication.

Therefore still their eyeballs shrink tormented
Back into their brains, because on their sense
Sunlight seems a blood-smear; night comes blood-black;
Dawn breaks open like a wound that bleeds afresh.
—Thus their heads wear this hilarious, hideous,
Awful falseness of set-smiling corpses.
—Thus their hands are plucking at each other;
Picking at the rope-knouts of their scourging;
Snatching after us who smote them, brother,
Pawing us who dealt them war and madness.

Edna St. Vincent Millay

(1892–1950)

Sorrow

Sorrow like a ceaseless rain
   Beats upon my heart.
People twist and scream in pain,—
Dawn will find them still again;
This has neither wax nor wane,
   Neither stop nor start.

People dress and go to town;
   I sit in my chair.
All my thoughts are slow and brown:
Standing up or sitting down
Little matters, or what gown
   Or what shoes I wear.

"I know a hundred ways to die"

I know a hundred ways to die.
I've often thought I'd try one:
Lie down beneath a motor truck
Some day when standing by one.

Or throw myself from off a bridge—
Except such things must be
So hard upon the scavengers
And men that clean the sea.

I know some poison I could drink.
I've often thought I'd taste it.
But mother bought it for the sink,
And drinking it would waste it.

～

Menses

(He speaks, but to himself, being aware how it is with her)

Think not I have not heard.
Well-fanged the double word
And well-directed flew.

I felt it. Down my side
Innocent as oil I see the ugly venom slide:
Poison enough to stiffen us both, and all our friends;
But I am not pierced, so there the mischief ends.

There is more to be said: I see it coiling;
The impact will be pain.
Yet coil; yet strike again.
You cannot riddle the stout mail I wove
Long since, of wit and love.

As for my answer . . . stupid in the sun
He lies, his fangs drawn:
I will not war with you.

You know how wild you are. You are willing to be turned
To other matters; you would be grateful, even.
You watch me shyly. I (for I have learned
More things than one in our few years together)
Chafe at the churlish wind, the unseasonable weather.

"Unseasonable?" you cry, with harsher scorn
Than the theme warrants; "Every year it is the same!
'Unseasonable!' they whine, these stupid peasants!—and never
   since they were born
Have they known a spring less wintry! Lord, the shame,
The crying shame of seeing a man no wiser than the beasts he feeds—
His skull as empty as a shell!"

("Go to. You are unwell.")

Such is my thought, but such are not my words.

"What is the name," I ask, "of those big birds
With yellow breast and low and heavy flight,
That make such mournful whistling?"

"Meadowlarks,"
You answer primly, not a little cheered.
"Some people shoot them." Suddenly your eyes are wet
And your chin trembles. On my breast you lean,
And sob most pitifully for all the lovely things that are not and
   have been.

"How silly I am!—and I know how silly I am!"
You say; "You are very patient. You are very kind.
I shall be better soon. Just Heaven consign and damn
To tedious Hell this body with its muddy feet in my mind!"

Dorothy Parker

(1893–1967)

Resume

Razors pain you;
Rivers are damp;
Acids stain you;
And drugs cause cramp.
Guns aren't lawful;
Nooses give;
Gas smells awful;
You might as well live.

Louise Bogan

(1897–1970)

Evening in the Sanitarium

The free evening fades, outside the windows fastened
    with decorative iron grilles.
The lamps are lighted; the shades drawn; the nurses are
    watching a little.
It is the hour of the complicated knitting on the safe bone
    needles; of the games of anagrams and bridge;
The deadly game of chess; the book held up like a mask.

The period of the wildest weeping, the fiercest delusion,
    is over.
The women rest their tired half-healed hearts; they are
    almost well.
Some of them will stay almost well always: the blunt-
    faced woman whose thinking dissolved
Under academic discipline; the manic-depressive girl
Now leveling off; one paranoiac afflicted with jealousy.
Another with persecution. Some alleviation has been
    possible.

O fortunate bride, who never again will become elated
    after childbirth!
O lucky older wife, who has been cured of feeling
    unwanted!
To the suburban railway station you will return, return,
To meet forever Jim home on the 5:35.
You will be again as normal and selfish and heartless as
    anybody else.

There is life left: the piano says it with its octave smile.
The soft carpets pad the thump and splinter of the
    suicide to be.
Everything will be splendid: the grandmother will not
    drink habitually.

The fruit salad will bloom on the plate like a bouquet
And the garden produce the blue-ribbon aquilegia.
The cats will be glad; the fathers feel justified; the
    mothers relieved.
The sons and husbands will no longer need to pay the bills.
Childhoods will be put away, the obscene nightmare abated.

At the ends of the corridors the baths are running.
Mrs. C. again feels the shadow of the obsessive idea.
Miss R. looks at the mantel-piece, which must mean
    something.

Hart Crane

(1899–1932)

The Idiot

Sheer over to the other side,—for see—
The boy straggling under those mimosas, daft
With squint lanterns in his head, and it's likely
Fumbling his sex. That's why those children laughed

In such infernal circles round his door
Once when he shouted, stretched in ghastly shape.
I hurried by. But back from the hot shore
Passed him again . . . He was alone, agape;

One hand dealt out a kite string, a tin can
The other tilted, peeled end clamped to eye.
That kite aloft—you should have watched him scan
Its course, though he'd clapped midnight to noon sky!

And since, through these hot barricades of green,
A Dios gracias, grac—I've heard his song
Above all reason lifting, halt serene—
My trespass vision shrinks to face his wrong.

(John Orley) Allen Tate

(1899–1979)

Ode to Fear

Let the day glare: O memory, your tread
Beats to the pulse of suffocating night—
Night peering from his dark but fire-lit head
Burns on the day his tense and secret light.

Now they dare not to gloss your savage dream,
O beast of the heart, those saints who cursed your name;
You are the current of the frozen stream,
Shadow invisible, ambushed and vigilant flame.

My eldest companion present in solitude,
Watch-dog of Thebes when the blind hero strove:
You, omniscient, at the cross-roads stood
When Laius, the slain dotard, drenched the grove.

Now to the eye of prophecy immune,
Fading and harried, you stalk us in the street
From the recesses of the August noon,
Alert world over, crouched on the air's feet.

You are our surety to immortal life,
God's hatred of the universal stain—
The heritage, O Fear, of ancient strife
Compounded with the tissue of the vein.

And I when all is said have seen your form
Most agile and most treacherous to the world
When, on a child's long day, a dry storm
Burst on the cedars, lit by the sun and hurled!

Anonymous

(published 1930)

from "Thoughts Suggested on a Thanksgiving Day Passed at the State Lunatic Asylum, Worcester, Mass., by a Patient"

Hark! 'tis the chapel bell!—its lively peal,
At early morn, wakes, from their slumbering beds,
The various members of this household band.
Forth to their several duties, each they hie—
The faithful *"Nurse,"* with beaming lamp in hand,
The healing potion from the "doctor" bears;
Which being administered, she speeds to arrange,
In order due, the frugal meal.—Meanwhile,
As, careful of her trust, she goes from room
To room, to inquire the health, each little want
To learn, the pleasant *"Supervisor's"* voice
Is heard.—The worthy *"Steward"* too, whose care
Unwearied, and whose generous deeds, have won
Him many a well deserved epithet
Of fame, himself betakes the building o'er
T' survey.—The clock strikes seven: the signal's given,
And now, with hair adjusted, person washed,
In neat attire, behold th' assembled group
Around the well set board; the pleasant word 's
Exchanged; the thoughts of many homeward turn,
Which utterance find in words of sad regret
At separation thus from those they love,
And in whose blest society they oft,
On day like this have swelled the thankful song.
Some cheerful, happy, look; while other some,
In listless reverie, seem mindful scarce
Of aught.—All now is life;—the breakfast o'er,
The cloth's removed, while brooms and brushes quick
Are plied, to sweep the gathered dust, t' restore
That perfect neatness, which is wont to reign
Within these walls. Here *order*, in its prime,
Presides, *system complete*, that which could be

Nought perfect more; for all in concert move,
With jarring seldom mix'd confusion ne'er.

The much loved *"Matron's"* gentle footstep's heard,
Whose tender sympathy by all is felt.
Is any sick? How carefully she strives
To soothe the pain, t' administer relief
And comfort as she can. Is any sad?
Her voice she lifts, each drooping heart to cheer.

Anon—the venerated *"Doctor's"* voice we list;
He, with his *"Aid,"* whose arduous labors none
Could better, few so well sustain, explores
The several wards.—None 'scapes their notice; *all*
Their kindness share. Each room, however lone,
Is lighted by their presence oft. For e'en
The raving maniac is not senseless all,
To tones of love and acts of mercy kind;
He has a *heart*, which has not ceased to throb
At deeds of pity, where he well can trace
The sympathetic tear; and long his mind,
Though broken, past repair, will yet retain
In fond remembrance, grateful thoughts like these,
And oft will speak, in eager terms of true
Affectionate regard and bland respect,
The name of *Dr. Woodward*, in whose heart,
He *feels* his interests dwell. For easily
He reads, marked in his very countenance,
So kind, so full of tenderness, his love
For poor unfortunates, who but for him,
E'en now, might in some dungeon lie in chains,
Exposed to cold, to hunger, and distress.
But here their comfort's sought: a snug warm room
Is theirs to occupy, while wholesome food
Is furnished, raiment clean, and all is done
Which human kindness can suggest, to make
Them happy here.

                              · · ·

'Tis six o'clock.———Again a summons to
The *"Hall."* For what? Not for the frolic dance,
The jovial song, the sparkling glass, but there

To renovate the sinking mind, to give
Vitality to such as lost appear
To all that interests. A season here
Is passed in rational delight: the sad,
The excited, both, their partners choose; and now,
At sound of viol sweet, and mellow flute,
Is opened the *"Thanksgiving Ball."* With what
Good order, time and step observed, the dance
Proceeds! Now oft a smile's observed, where both
Despondency and gloom had long been wont
To shade the countenance. Often, here, the spark
Of hope revives, and by degrees is fanned
To flame, which many months had dormant lain,
And seemed well nigh extinguished. Who can doubt
The use of means like these, or grateful fail
To feel, that God has given in mercy thus
To the discreet physician, to devise
Such skilful schemes, and to them grants success?
For well we know, that effort all is vain,
Without our Heavenly Father's blessing given.

. . .

Anonymous

(published 1930)

Awakening

from: *Poetry of the Insane* (Charles Mayos, editor)

The hue of sorrow everywhere
The jagged rocks seem marble tombs,
Yet through the barren waste way over there,
A lily blooms.

As up the rugged heights revealed,
I creep, and deem the world as wrong;
A singer trills above the love unsealed,
His mating song.

I pierce the gloom with purer eyes,
For here I know that Heaven is—
I yield my empty self and realize
These are all His.

Mendocino State Hospital,
Talmage, California

The Snow

The snow, the snow, the beautiful snow!
   Snow on the window ledge, above and below,
Snow on the hedges, dead leaves peeping out,
   Snow hanging down from the old rain-spout.

How it scurries, hurries and flurries,
   How it makes us forget our worries,
Flakes in tiny, beautiful form
   Stars, angles and hexagons.

Snow in the park trees and band-stand,
   A white mantle o'er all the land,
Snow in the flower beds—like frosted cake
   Old thoughts come, makes your heartache.

The wind blows cold, the snow it whirls,
   Jumping right into our permanent curls,
Soft and feathery, and light as a spray,
   Gosh! how beautiful, if you don't care what you
      say.

Now a fierce gust whirling below,
   Hold down your dress! Naughty, naughty snow!
Look kind of innocent—make a snow ball,
   Peck the old "hen" nurse, standing by the wall.

Snow in the bird's nest among the dead leaves,
   Fluffy cream whip, hanging o'er the eaves,
How last summer's leaves cling and quiver
   Everything is cold and dead, how it makes me
      shiver.

And my old blue moods, they're always there,
   Some bring thoughts of home and I cry,
Now look what I am and where,
   Please God, let me die!

East Moline State Hospital,
East Moline, Illinois

The Cure

You laughed at me, called me a fool,
    When I told you of long nights awake.
You said you would listen no more
    To the vows that I took for love's sake.

You tortured me heart for a cure,
    As only a wanton can do.
But you didn't cure me of love;
    You only cured me of you.

New Jersey State Hospital,
Greystone Park, New Jersey

Richard David Comstock

(published 1930)

Always Like This

I want to get well, but I can't, it seems,
And I'm still disturbed in my restless dreams,
And I just can't catch the sunlight's beams.
    Will it always be like this?

There's something bothers me all night.
It hectors, taunts till the morning's light,
And the mirror shows me a sorry sight.
    Will I always look like this?

I try to do just as the doctors say
And do it all in the proper way,
But still I drag on thru' listless days.
    Will all days be like this?

But one thing sure, there's room for a grave
On the old home ranch where the free
        winds rave,
And its one long rest, with sorrow saved,
    Then it will not be like this.

I'm sick of the hustling to and fro,
And I want to go where there is no woe,
But I don't dare tell the doctor so,
    That things are so amiss,

For he'd give me a funny look,
And write me up in a black-bound book
Where the suicidal notes are took,
    I'd be much worse off than this.

Stanley Kunitz

(1905–2006)

The Portrait

My mother never forgave my father
for killing himself,
especially at such an awkward time
and in a public park,
that spring
when I was waiting to be born.
She locked his name
in her deepest cabinet
and would not let him out,
though I could hear him thumping.
When I came down from the attic
with the pastel portrait in my hand
of a long-lipped stranger
with a brave moustache
and deep brown level eyes,
she ripped it into shreds
without a single word
and slapped me hard.
In my sixty-fourth year
I can feel my cheek
still burning.

Theodore Roethke

(1908–1963)

In a Dark Time

In a dark time, the eye begins to see,
I meet my shadow in the deepening shade;
I hear my echo in the echoing wood—
A lord of nature weeping to a tree.
I live between the heron and the wren,
Beasts of the hill and serpents of the den.

What's madness but nobility of soul
At odds with circumstance? The day's on fire!
I know the purity of pure despair,
My shadow pinned against a sweating wall.
That place among the rocks—is it a cave,
Or winding path? The edge is what I have.

A steady storm of correspondences!
A night flowing with birds, a ragged moon,
And in broad day the midnight come again!
A man goes far to find out what he is—
Death of the self in a long, tearless night,
All natural shapes blazing unnatural light.

Dark, dark my light, and darker my desire.
My soul, like some heat-maddened summer fly,
Keeps buzzing at the sill. Which I is *I*?
A fallen man, I climb out of my fear.
The mind enters itself, and God the mind,
And one is One, free in the tearing wind.

Her Longing

Before this longing,
I lived serene as a fish,
At one with the plants in the pond,
The mare's tail, the floating frogbit,
Among my eight-legged friends,
Open like a pool, a lesser parsnip,
Like a leech, looping myself along,
A bug-eyed edible one,
A mouth like a stickleback,—
A thing quiescent!

But now—
The wild stream, the sea itself cannot contain me:
I dive with the black hag, the cormorant,
Or walk the pebbly shore with the humpbacked heron,
Shaking out my catch in the morning sunlight,
Or rise with the gar-eagle, the great-winged condor.
Floating over the mountains,
Pitting my breast against the rushing air,
A phoenix, sure of my body,
Perpetually rising out of myself,
My wings hovering over the shorebirds,
Or beating against the black clouds of the storm,
Protecting the sea-cliffs.

Lines Upon Leaving a Sanitarium

Self-contemplation is a curse
That makes an old confusion worse.

Recumbency is unrefined
And leads to errors in the mind.

Long gazing at the ceiling will
In time induce a mental ill.

The mirror tells some truth, but not
Enough to merit constant thought.

He who himself begins to loathe
Grows sick in flesh and spirit both.

Dissection is a virtue when
It operates on other men.

Elizabeth Bishop

(1911–1979)

Visits to Saint Elizabeths

This is the house of Bedlam.

This is the man
that lies in the house of Bedlam.

This is the time
of the tragic man
that lies in the house of Bedlam.

This is a wristwatch
telling the time
of the talkative man
that lies in the house of Bedlam.

This is a sailor
wearing the watch
that tells the time
of the honored man
that lies in the house of Bedlam.

This is the roadstead all of board
reached by the sailor
wearing the watch
that tells the time
of the old, brave man
that lies in the house of Bedlam.

These are the years and the walls of the ward,
the winds and clouds of the sea of board
sailed by the sailor
wearing the watch
that tells the time
of the cranky man
that lies in the house of Bedlam.

This is a Jew in a newspaper hat
that dances weeping down the ward
over the creaking sea of board
beyond the sailor
winding his watch
that tells the time
of the cruel man
that lies in the house of Bedlam.

This is a world of books gone flat.
This is a Jew in a newspaper hat
that dances weeping down the ward
over the creaking sea of board
of the batty sailor
that winds his watch
that tells the time
of the busy man
that lies in the house of Bedlam.

This is a boy that pats the floor
to see if the world is there, is flat,
for the widowed Jew in the newspaper hat
that dances weeping down the ward
waltzing the length of a weaving board
by the silent sailor
that hears his watch
that ticks the time
of the tedious man
that lies in the house of Bedlam.

These are the years and the walls and the door
that shut on a boy that pats the floor
to feel if the world is there and flat.
This is a Jew in a newspaper hat
that dances joyfully down the ward
into the parting seas of board
past the staring sailor
that shakes his watch
that tells the time
of the poet, the man
that lies in the house of Bedlam.

This is the soldier home from the war.
These are the years and the walls and the door
that shut on a boy that pats the floor
to see if the world is round or flat.
This is a Jew in a newspaper hat
that dances carefully down the ward,
walking the plank of a coffin board
with the crazy sailor
that shows his watch
that tells the time
of the wretched man
that lies in the house of Bedlam.

J. V. (James Vincent) Cunningham

(1911–1985)

from Interview with Doctor Drink

I have a fifth of therapy
In the house, and transference there.
Doctor, there's not much wrong with me,
Only a sick rattlesnake somewhere

In the house, if it be there at all,
But the lithe mouth is coiled. The shapes
Of door and window move. I call.
What is it that pulls down the drapes,

Disheveled and exposed? Your rye
Twists in my throat: intimacy
Is like hard liquor. Who but I
Coil there and squat, and pay your fee?

Delmore Schwartz

(1913–1966)

from "The Studies of Narcissus"

. . .

The mind is a city like London,
Smoky and populous: it is a capital
Like Rome, ruined and eternal,
Marked by the monuments which no one
Now remembers. For the mind, like Rome, contains
Catacombs, aqueducts, amphitheatres, palaces,
Churches and equestrian statues, fallen, broken or soiled.
The mind possesses and is possessed by all the ruins
Of every haunted, hunted generation's celebration.

. . .

I waited like obsession in solitude:
The sun's white terror tore and roared at me,
The moonlight, almond white, at night,
Whether awake or sleeping, arrested me
And sang, softly, haunted, unlike the sun
But as the sun. Withheld from me or took away
Despair or peace, making me once more
With thought of what had never been before—
—The others were the despots of despair—

The river's freshness sailed from unknown sources—

. . . They snickered giggled, laughed aloud at last,
They mocked and marvelled at the statue which was
A caricature, as strained and stiff, and yet
A statue of self-love!—since self-love was
To them, truly my true love, how, then, was I a stillness
    of nervousness
So nervous a caricature: did they suppose
Self-love was unrequited, or betrayed?

They thought I had fallen in love with my own face,
And this belief became the night-like obstacle
To understanding all my unbroken suffering,
My studious soft-regard, the pain of hope,
The torment of possibility:
How then could I have expected them to see me
As I saw myself, within my gaze, or see
That being thus seemed as a toad, a frog, a wen, a mole.
Knowing their certainty that I was only
A monument, a monster who had fallen in love
With himself alone, how could I have
Told them what was in me, within my heart, trembling,
    and passionate
Within the labyrinth and caves of my mind, which is
Like every mind partly or wholly hidden from itself?
The words for what is in my heart and in my mind
Do not exist: But I must seek and search to find
Amid the vines and orchards of the vivid world of day
Approximate images, imaginary parallels
For what is in my heart and dark within my mind:
Comparisons and mere metaphors: for all
Of them are substitutes, both counterfeit and vague:
They are, at most, deceptive resemblances,
False in their very likeness, like the sons
Who are alike and kin and more unlike and false
Because they seem the fathers' very self: but each one is
—Although begotten by the same forbears—himself,
The unique self, each one is unique, like every other one,
And everything, older or younger, nevertheless
A passionate nonesuch who before has been.
Do you hear, do you see? Do you understand me now, and how
The words for what is my heart do not exist?

. . .

from *Genesis*, Book II

. . .

The main thing: Atlantic boy, is to see Life,
To see it as a progress and waste of days,
        that is, as a story,
In which are certain scenes which seem to show
        all that was there a while,
The glittering attractions of dignity and pleasure. . . .

"The mind is the greatest tourist, never at home,
And hence freely we pass through the places where Life
        has agreed or agonized,
So we go on, seldom satisfied even a while:

But when we think of that Consciousness which sees all,
When then our minds like larks at heaven's gate sing,
Sing on, sing out
        our endless memory and hope of all things!"

"Nothing is left unsaid, no shame forgiven!
Nothing that I escape in common pity,"
Cried Hershey Green,
        "Who knows so much about me,
Yet does not let me fly from agony,
Except, like tortured men to convalesce
Before the rack once more is placed upon
His hands, his mind, his pride, his private parts!
—All of the sordor that my life has known,
Every disorder, together or alone!
I take my guilt! I know it very well:
Was I the only one like that? Do they,
Like me, rehearse it over and over again?
        all of it, every shame?
Whether they do or not, *I wish to die!*"

. . .

"Not God himself can quite destroy the Past!
What's his forgiveness then? All men, Macbeth!"
So cried the tortured boy, crying for death!

220

"'O Death, great captain, lift anchor!
                    it is time!'
And lift away this passionate ruined man:
This guilty boy show how *he* does not die,
This boy is but one act of his, in dying . . .
                    Will move with you!
This gulf, Atlantic boy, will move with you,
As Pascal and Baudelaire, henceforth—
You will fear Death as one fears a great height
Full of vague horror leading who knows where? . . ."

"You will see the infinite at every window,
Desiring always insensibility,
Which is your wish throughout this shameful night . . .
—Across the depth of your nights, God's knowing hand
Will draw more nightmares, greater terror
                    and horror,
Without an exit and without conclusion—"

"Thus all is a gulf,—'action, desire, hope,'
Language and thought. Silence is under all,
Appalling and empty space surrounds you now:
You lie in the coffin of your character,
Trapped by each effort to escape from it,
Just like a fly caught in a treacherous sweet—"

                    . . .

John Berryman

(1914–1972)

Dreamsongs 172

Your face broods from my table, Suicide.
Your force came on like a torrent toward the end
of agony and wrath.
You were christened in the beginning Sylvia Plath
and changed that name for Mrs Hughes and bred
and went on round the bend

till the oven seemed the proper place for you.
I brood upon your face, the geography of grief,
hooded, till I allow
again your resignation from us now
though the screams of orphaned children fix me anew.
Your torment here was brief,

long falls your exit all repeatingly,
a poor exemplum, one more suicide,
to stack upon the others
till stricken Henry with his sisters & brothers
suddenly gone pauses to wonder why he
alone breasts the wronging tide.

Randall Jarrell

(1914–1965)

In the Ward: The Sacred Wood

The trees rise from the darkness of the world.
The little trees, the paper grove,
Stand woodenly, a sigh of earth,
Upon the table by this bed of life
Where I have lain so long: until at last
I find a Maker for them, and forget
Who cut them from their cardboard, brushed
A bird on each dark, fretted bough.
But the birds think and are still.
The thunder mutters to them from the hills
My knees make by the rainless Garden.
If the grove trembles with the fan
And makes, at last, its little flapping song
That wanders to me over the white flood
On which I float enchanted—shall I fall?
A bat jerks to me from the ragged limb
And hops across my shudder with its leaf
Of curling paper: have the waters gone?
Is the nurse damned who looked on my nakedness?
The sheets stretch like the wilderness
Up which my fingers wander, the sick tribes,
To a match's flare, a rain or bush of fire
Through which the devil trudges, coal by coal,
With all his goods; and I look absently
And am not tempted.
Death scratches feebly at this husk of life
In which I lie unchanging, Sin despairs
Of my dull works; and I am patient . . .
A third of all the angels, in the wars
Of God against the Angel, took no part
And were to God's will neither enemies
Nor followers, but lay in doubt:
             but lie in doubt.

There is no trade here for my life.
The lamb naps in the crêche, but will not die.
The halo strapped upon the head
Of the doctor who stares down my throat
And thinks, "Die, then; I shall not die"—
Is this the glitter of the cruze of oil
Upon the locks of that Anointed One
Who gazes, dully, from the leafless tree
Into the fixed eyes of Elohim?
I have made the Father call indifferently
To a body, to the Son of Man:
"It is finished." And beneath the coverlet
My limbs are swaddled in their sleep, and shade
Flows from the cave beyond the olives, falls
Into the garden where no messenger
Comes to gesture, "Go"—to whisper, "He is gone."

The trees rise to me from the world
That made me, I call to the grove
That stretches inch on inch without one God:
"I have unmade you, now; but I must die."

Weldon Kees

(1914–1955)

from "The Fall of the Magicians"

4

No sound except the beating of a drum
Is heard along this walled-in corridor.
"Time will go by," we heard; "no messages will come."

The guests seem sad without their opium.
They stare at me and talk about the war.
There is not sound except the beating of a drum.

They want a different noise; like me, they thumb
Through heavy books we keep behind the door.
"Time will go by," we heard; "no messages will come."

Noise with complexity, however glum,
Might give some clue to what there is in store,
But there's no sound except the beating of a drum.

A few wear beards, or sleep all day, while some
Have grown quite philosophical. Some pace the floor.
"Time will go by," we heard; "no messages will come."

I think it is our hearts. Each paralyzed and numb
With waiting. Yet what is it we are waiting for?
No sound except the beating of a drum?
"Time will go by," we heard. "No messages will come."

The Clinic

Light in the cage like burning foil
At noon; and I am caught
With all the other cats that howl
And dance and spit, lashing their tails
When the doctors turn the current on.
The ceiling fries. Waves shimmer from the floor
Where hell spreads thin between the bars.
And then a switch snaps off and it is over
For another day. Close up. Go home.
Calcium chloride, a milligram
Or so, needled into the brain, close to
The infundibulum. Sometimes we sleep for weeks.
Report
From Doctor Edwards: sixteen tests (five women, fourteen men).
Results are far from positive. Static ataxia,
Blood pressure, tapping, visual acuity. A Mrs. Wax
Could not recall a long ride in a Chevrolet
From Jersey to her home in Forest Hills. Fatigue
Reported by a few. These smoky nights
My eyes feel dry and raw; I tire
After twenty hours without sleep. Performance
At a lower ebb.—The lights
Have flickered and gone out.
There is a sound like winter in the streets.
Vide Master,
Muzie, Brown and Parker on the hypoplastic heart.
Culpin stressed the psychogenic origin. DaCosta
Ruled out syphilis. If we follow Raines and Kolb,
We follow Raines and Kolb.—It's only a sort of wound,
From one of the wars, that opens up occasionally.
Signs of desiccation, but very little pain.

I followed Raines and Kolb, in that dark backward,
Seeking a clue; yet in that blackness, hardly a drop
Of blood within me did not shudder. Mouths without hands,
Eyes without light, my tongue dry, intolerable
Thirst. And then we came into that room
Where a world of cats danced, spat, and howled
Upon a burning plate.—And I was home.

Dylan Thomas

(1914–1953)

Out of the Sighs

Out of the sighs a little comes,
But not of grief, for I have knocked down that
Before the agony; the spirit grows,
Forgets, and cries;
A little comes, is tasted and found good;
All could not disappoint;
There must, be praised, some certainty,
If not of loving well, then not,
And that is true after perpetual defeat.

After such fighting as the weakest know,
There's more than dying;
Lose the great pains or stuff the wound,
He'll ache too long
Through no regret of leaving woman waiting
For her soldier stained with split words
That spill such acrid blood.

Were that enough, enough to ease the pain,
Feeling regret when this is wasted
That made me happy in the sun,
How much was happy while it lasted,
Were vagueness enough and the sweet lies plenty,
The hollow words could bear all suffering
And cure me of ills.

Were that enough, bone, blood, and sinew,
The twisted brain, the fair-formed loin,
Groping for matter under the dog's plate,
Man should be cured of distemper.
For all there is to give I offer:
Crumbs, barn, and halter.

Robert Lowell

(1917–1977)

Visitors

To no good
they enter at angles and on the run—
two black verticals are suddenly four
ambulance drivers in blue serge,
or the police doing double-duty.
They comb our intimate, messy bedroom,
scrutinize worksheets
illegible with second-thoughts,
then shed them in their stride,
as if they owned the room. They do.
They crowd me and scatter—inspecting
my cast-off clothes for clues?
They are fat beyond the call of duty—
with jocose civility,
they laugh at everything I say:
"Yesterday I was thirty-two, a threat
to the establishment because I was young."
The bored woman sergeant
is amused by the tiger-toothed samurai
grinning on a Japanese hanging—
"What would it cost? Where could I buy one?"

I can see through the moonlit dark;
on the grassy London square,
black cows ruminate in uniform,
lowing routinely like a chainsaw.
My visitors are good beef, they too make
one falsely feel the earth is solid,
as they hurry to secretly telephone
from their ambulance. Click, click, click,
goes the red, blue, and white light
burning with aristocratic negligence—
so much busywork.

When they regroup in my room, I know
their eyes have never left their watches.
"Come on, sir." "Easy, sir."
"Dr. Brown will be here in ten minutes, sir."
Instead, a metal chair unfolds into a stretcher.
I lie secured there, but for my skipping mind.
They keep bustling.
"Where you are going, Professor,
you won't need your Dante."
What will I need there?
Is that a handcuff rattling in a pocket?

I follow my own removal,
stiffly, gratefully even, but without feeling.
Why has my talkative
teasing tongue stopped talking?
My detachment must be paid for,
tomorrow will be worse than today,
heaven and hell will be the same—
to wait in foreboding
without the nourishment of drama . . .
assuming, then as now,
this didn't happen to me—
my little strip of eternity.

Waking in the Blue

The night attendant, a B.U. sophomore,
rouses from the mare's-nest of his drowsy head
propped on *The Meaning of Meaning.*
He catwalks down our corridor.
Azure day
makes my agonized blue window bleaker.
Crows maunder on the petrified fairway.
Absence! My hearts grows tense

as though a harpoon were sparring for the kill.
(This is the house for the "mentally ill.")

What use is my sense of humour?
I grin at Stanley, now sunk in his sixties,
once a Harvard all-American fullback,
(if such were possible!)
still hoarding the build of a boy in his twenties,
as he soaks, a ramrod
with a muscle of a seal
in his long tub,
vaguely urinous from the Victorian plumbing.
A kingly granite profile in a crimson gold-cap,
worn all day, all night,
he thinks only of his figure,
of slimming on sherbert and ginger ale—
more cut off from words than a seal.
This is the way day breaks in Bowditch Hall at McLean's;
the hooded night lights bring out "Bobbie,"
Porcellian '29,
a replica of Louis XVI
without the wig—
redolent and roly-poly as a sperm whale,
as he swashbuckles about in his birthday suit
and horses at chairs.

These victorious figures of bravado ossified young.

In between the limits of day,
hours and hours go by under the crew haircuts
and slightly too little nonsensical bachelor twinkle
of the Roman Catholic attendants.
(There are no Mayflower
screwballs in the Catholic Church.)
After a hearty New England breakfast,
I weigh two hundred pounds
this morning. Cock of the walk,
I strut in my turtle-necked French sailor's jersey
before the metal shaving mirrors,
and see the shaky future grow familiar
in the pinched, indigenous faces
of these thoroughbred mental cases,

twice my age and half my weight.
We are all old-timers,
each of us holds a locked razor.

Home After Three Months Away

Gone now the baby's nurse,
a lioness who ruled the roost
and made the Mother cry.
She used to tie
gobbets of porkrind in bowknots of gauze—
three months they hung like soggy toast
on our eight foot magnolia tree,
and helped the English sparrows
weather a Boston winter.

Three months, three months!
Is Richard now himself again?
Dimpled with exaltation,
my daughter holds her levee in the tub.
Our noses rub,
each of us pats a stringy lock of hair—
they tell me nothing's gone.
Though I am forty-one,
not forty now, the time I put away
was child's play. After thirteen weeks
my child still dabs her cheeks
to start me shaving. When
we dress her in her sky-blue corduroy,
she changes to a boy,
and floats my shaving brush
and washcloth in the flush. . . .
Dearest I cannot loiter here
in lather like a polar bear.

Recuperating, I neither spin nor toil.
Three stories down below,
a choreman tends our coffin's length of soil,
and seven horizontal tulips blow.
Just twelve months ago,
these flowers were pedigreed
imported Dutchmen; no no one need
distinguish them from weed.
Bushed by the late spring snow,
they cannot meet
another year's snowballing enervation.
I keep no rank nor station.
Cured, I am frizzled, stale and small.

Unwanted

Too late, all shops closed—
I alone here tonight on *Antabuse*,
surrounded only by iced white wine and beer,
like a sailor dying of thirst on the Atlantic—
one sip of alcohol might be death,
death for joy.
Yet in this tempting leisure,
good thoughts drive out bad;
causes for my misadventure, considered
for forty years too obvious to name,
come jumbling out
to give my simple autobiography a plot.

I read an article on a friend,
as if recognizing my obituary:
"Though his mother loved her son consumingly,
she lacked a really affectionate nature;
so he always loved what he missed."
This was John Berryman's mother, not mine.

Alas, I can only tell my own story—
talking to myself, or reading, or writing,
or fearlessly holding back nothing from a friend,
who believes me for a moment
to keep up conversation.

I was surer, wasn't I, once . . .
and had flashes when I first found
a humor for myself in images,
farfetched misalliance
that made evasion a revelation?

Dr. Merrill Moore, the family psychiatrist,
had unpresentable red smudge eyebrows,
and no infirmity for tact—
in his conversation or letters,
each phrase a new
paragraph,
implausible as the million
sonnets he rhymed into his dictaphone,
or dashed on windshield writing-pads,
while waiting out a stoplight—
scattered pearls, some true.
Dead he is still a mystery,
once a crutch to writers in crisis.
I am two-tongued, I will not admit
his Tennessee rattling saved my life.
Did he become mother's lover
and prey
by rescuing her from me?
He was thirteen years her junior . . .
When I was in college, he said, "You know
you were an unwanted child?"
Was he striking my parents to help me?
I shook him off the scent by pretending
anyone is unwanted in a medical sense—
lust our only father . . . and yet
in that world where an only child
was a scandal—
unwanted before I am?

That year Carl Jung said to mother in Zurich,
"If your son is as you have described him,
he is an incurable schizophrenic."

In 1916
father on sea-duty, mother with child
in one house with her affectionate mother-in-law,
unconsuming, already consumptive . . .
bromidic to mother . . . Mother,
I must not blame you for carrying me in you
on your brisk winter lunges across
the desperate, refusey Staten Island beaches,
their good view skyscrapers on Wall Street . . .
for yearning seaward, far from any home, and saying,
"I wish I were dead, I wish I were dead."
Unforgivable for a mother to tell her child—
but you wanted me to share your good fortune,
perhaps, by recapturing the disgust of those walks;
your credulity assumed we survived,
while weaklings fell with the dead and dying.

That consuming love,
woman's everlasting *cri de coeur*,
"When you have a child of your own, you'll know."
Her dowry for her children . . .

One thing is certain—compared with my wives,
mother was stupid. Was she?
Some would not have judged so—
among them, her alcoholic patients,
those raconteurish, old Boston young men,
whose fees, late in her life
and to everyone's concern,
she openly halved with Merrill Moore.
Since time out of mind, mother's gay hurting
assessments of enemies and intimates
had made her a formidable character
to her "reading club," seven ladies,
who since her early twenties
met once a week through winters
in their sitting rooms for confidence and tea—

she couldn't read a book . . .
How many of her statements began with,
But Papá always said or Oh Bobby . . .
if she Bryonized her father and son,
she saw her husband as a valet sees through a master.

She was stupider than my wife . . .
When I was three months,
I rocked back and forth howling
for weeks, for weeks each hour . . .
Then I found the thing I loved most
was the anorexia Christ
swinging on Nellie's gaudy rosary.
It disappeared, I said nothing,
but mother saw me poking strips of paper
down a floor-grate to the central heating.
"Oh Bobby, do you want to set us on fire?"
"Yes . . . that's where Jesus is." I smiled.

Is the one unpardonable sin
our fear of not being wanted?
For this, will mother go on cleaning house
for eternity, and making it unlivable?
Is getting well ever an art,
or art a way to get well?

Robert Edward Duncan

(1919–1988)

Songs of An Other

If there were another . . .

if there were an other
person I am he would
be heavy as the shadow

in a dying tree.   The light
thickens into water
welling up to liven

whose eyes? who hides his mother
behind him mirrord in his
bride's gaze   when the flame

darkens the music as he plays?
for I am here the Master of a Sonata
meant for the early evening

when in late Spring
the day begins to linger on
and we do not listen to the news

but let the wars and crises go
revering strife in a sound of our own,
a momentary leading of a tone

toward a conflicting possibility and then
fury so slowd down it lapses
into the sweetening melancholy of

a minor key, hovering toward refrain
it yet refrains from,   I come into
the being of this other me,

exquisitely alone,   everything   about the voice
has it own solitude the speech
addresses and, still accompanied,

kindled thruout by you,   every thought
of bride and groom comes to,
        my other

cannot keep his strangeness separate
there is such a presence of "home"
in every room I come to.

Howard Nemerov

(1920–1991)

To D——, Dead by Her Own Hand

My dear, I wonder if before the end
You ever thought about a children's game—
I'm sure you must have played it too—in which
You ran along a narrow garden wall
Pretending it to be a mountain ledge
So steep a snowy darkness fell away
On either side to deeps invisible;
And when you felt your balance being lost
You jumped because you feared to fall, and thought
For only an instant: that was when I died.

That was a life ago. And now you've gone,
Who would no longer play the grown-ups' game
Where, balanced on the ledge above the dark,
You go on running and don't look down,
Nor ever jump because you fear to fall.

Hayden Carruth

(1921–)

from "**The Asylum**"

1

I came to this place one November day.
Mauve walls rose up then tranquilly, and still
Must rise to wind-burned eyes that way—
Old brickwork on a hill,
Surfaces of impunity beneath a gray
And listed sky. Yet I could read dismay
There rightward in a twisted beech
Whose nineteen leaves were glittering, each
A tear in a rigid eye caught in the pale
Deep-pouring wind. Now these walls
Are thin against the dense insistent gale,
No good when the wind talks in our halls,
Useless at night when these high window bars
Catch every whisper of wind that comes and falls,
Speaking, across my catacomb of stars.

. . .

4

I hurt. Hungrier flowers try my rank ground.
Indelible, one drifts across Japan,
Rooted as if its stem were wound
Into the heart of a man.
A crumpling sky, a blurted dawn—the sound
Of history burst the years and history drowned.
We lived. An aftersilence fell
Like a wave flooding the plains of hell,
For what word matters? Pity? Shame? The roots
Try my breast-cage, my bone
Gleams in the rot. I hear you, sir, cahoots
Calling from many a dolmen stone,
Murther, murther! Come on then, jacket me,

A flawed mind's failing. Look, the petals blown
On an idle wind, far, far out to sea!

   5

But once winds lightened, freshening fair from the West.
Hayscent, grandfather told me, filled the plain.
Then came the Great Man, voice possessed,
Broad brow and flashing mane,
Chanting the silver words of labor blest,
Deliverance come for God's folk all oppressed.
And the city at the prairie edge
Rises to meet him. Poets pledge
His name to glory, sweet locust blooms in the park.
"Onward!" And triumph fills
Men's eyes. (Not who, but that he came.) The dark
Is fading. See, the sunlight spills
Like silver down the street. Onward! How slow
The years have been. And onward! Freedom wills
The day. (But this all happened long ago.)

      . . .

   7

What does this wind say, plunging upon the land,
Torrents sinuous and thick? Shall
A long wind make me understand
One separable from all?
Ethics is not a study I had planned.
At the beginning is one cruel command:
Save thou thyself. But where? Dear crowd,
My dear little mad folk, cry loud,
Cry long, add your beseeching to this wind!
For it is a curious blast,
Both full and faint, as if my ears were dinned
By pulses not my own, but past.
Dusk, and the Troy fires wink below our hill.
And here we came to search the self at last,
And here the long wind comes, and comes to kill.

      . . .

   9

But if the wind should fall and silence spread
Like nightward dimness rising underseas,

Muffling many a fervid head,
Stilling the quick-tongued trees,
Stagnation creeping, loathed, in board and bed,
The weed, the bone, the dust, the spider's thread,
If nerve-song were suppressed to quell
Our quick wise hurting, if a smell
Of sleep-rot issued from us, black slime boiled
From our close scaly wall,
Water clotted and air's befoulment coiled
On each lost creature that could crawl
Apart beneath the mountainous dung-soft sky,
If this should be and if the wind should fall,
Could sane men live? Dear friends, could madmen die?

10

I came to this place one November day.
The winter deepened. Then at last came March,
Then May, and now another May,
Our outdoor season. A larch,
Of graceful habit, mounts its green display,
And we have almost nothing left to say.
Motley despondent pigeons pass
Like tick and tock across the grass.
The nurse assigned to govern shuffleboard
Is continually amazed,
Being young and pretty. The male attendants hoard
Their tedium like whiskey, poised
For anything. Up where the roofs are pearled
By sunlight, an arrow turns forever, seized
In our four winds, pointing across the world.

11

This nation was asylum when we came
On sea-qualms heaving west in wind-drenched ships
And found our plenty. But the home
We built here in these strips
Of wilderness could not resist the storm
That trailed us. It foundered like a tomb
Whose broken walls cannot protect
The dead from the toothy wind of fact.
Always this breaking. And is not the whole earth
Asylum? Is mankind

241

In refuge? Here is where we fled in birth.
Yet what we fled from we shall find,
It fills us now. And we shall search the air,
Turning drained eyes along the wind, as blind
Men do, but never find asylum here.

12

Then ultimately asylum is the soul.
Reason curls like a nut in wrinkled sleep,
And here, here on this windy knoll,
Our house was built to keep
One private semblance where we conceive our role.
Thus when our solemn inspectors come to stroll
The shadeless halls, our wives and friends,
We seldom mention how the winds
Shriek in their mouths. Gradually we feel
More natural, we try
To sink like the silent leaves that slide and reel
In anguish down the windy sky.
Sometimes it works. Sometimes we find out then
Our tiny irreducible selves. We die.
And after that we die again, again.

. . .

Lines Written in an Asylum

Lost sweetheart, how our memories creep
Like chidden hounds, and come to reap
All fawningly their servient due,
Their tax of pity and of rue,
So that my hope of sanity
Like sternness dies and falls from me.
The day I build with plotted hours
To stand apart is mine, not ours.

Its joyless business is my cure;
Stern and alone, I may endure.
But memory though it slumber wakes,
And deep in the mind its havoc makes.
A distant baying reels and swells
And floods the night, and so dispels
My hardness; hours dissolve and fall;
My loss is double: you, then all.
Dearest, are you so unaware?
For here, in mine, your senses share
These broken hours and tumbled days
That are no longer mine. Your ways,
The body's blossoms, breast and eye,
The soft songs of your hands, the shy
And quick amusement of your smile—
My constant losses, these beguile
All my new bravery away.
If you have gone, why do you stay?
If here, then why have we no ease?
Loss is a blindness that still sees,
A handless love that touches still.
Loss is a ravage of the will.
And the incontinence of loss,
Mad loneliness, turns all to dross,
Love to a raging discontent
And self to a shabby tenement.
The mind is hapless, torn by dreams
Where all becoming only seems
A false, impossible return
To a world I labor to unlearn.

from **"Ontological Episode of the Asylum"**

The boobyhatch's bars, the guards, the nurses,
The illimitable locks and keys are all arranged

To thwart the hand that continually rehearses
Its ending stroke and raise a barricade
Against destruction-seeking resolution.
Many of us in there would have given all
(But we had nothing) for one small razor blade
Or seventy grains of the comforting amytal.

So I went down in the attitude of prayer,
Yes, to my knees on the cold floor of my cell,
Humped in a corner, a bird with a broken wing,
And asked and asked as fervently and well
As I could guess to do for light in the mists
Of death, until I learned God doesn't care.
Not only that, he doesn't care at all,
One way or the other. That is why he exists.

Philip Larkin

(1922–1985)

Neurotics

No one gives you a thought, as day by day
You drag your feet, clay-thick with misery.
None think how stalemate in you grinds away,
Holding your spinning wheels an inch too high
To bite on earth. The mind, it's said, is free:
But not your minds, They, rusted stiff, admit
Only what will accuse or horrify,
Like slot-machines only bent pennies fit.

So year by year your tense unfinished faces
Sink further from the light. No one pretends
To want to help you now. For interest passes
Always towards the young and more insistent,
And skirts locked rooms where a hired darkness ends
Your long defence against the non-existent.

Anthony Hecht

(1923–2004)

A Deep Breath at Dawn

Morning has come at last. The rational light
Discovers even the humblest thing that yearns
For heaven; from its scaled and shadeless height,
Figures its difficult way among the ferns,
Nests in the trees, and is ambitious to warm
The chilled vein, and to light the spider's thread
With modulations hastening to a storm
Of the full spectrum, rushing from red to red.
I have watched its refinements since the dawn,
When, at the birdcall, all the ghosts were gone.

The wolf, the fig tree, and the woodpecker
Were sacred once to Undertaker Mars;
Honor was done in Rome to that home-wrecker
Whose armor and whose ancient, toughened scars
Made dance the very meat of Venus' heart,
And hot her ichor, and immense her eyes,
Till his rough ways and her invincible art
Locked and laid low their shining, tangled thighs.
My garden yields his fig tree, even now
Bearing heraldic fruit at every bough.

Someone I have not seen for six full years
Might pass this garden through, and might pass by
The oleander bush, the bitter pears
Unfinished by the sun, with only an eye
For the sun-speckled shade of the fig tree,
And shelter in its gloom, and raise his hand
For tribute and for nourishment (for he
Was once entirely at the god's command)
But that his nature, being all undone,
Cannot abide the clarity of the sun.

Morning deceived him those six years ago.
Morning swam in the pasture, being all green
And yellow, and the swallow coiled in slow
Passage of dials and spires above the scene
Cluttered with dandelions, near the fence
Where the hens strutted redheaded and wreathed
With dark, imponderable chicken sense,
Hardly two hundred yards from where he breathed,
And where, from their declamatory roosts,
The cocks cried brazenly against all ghosts.

Warmth in the milling air, the warmth of blood;
The dampness of the earth; the forest floor
Of fallen needles, the dried and creviced mud,
Lay matted and caked with sunlight, and the war
Seemed elsewhere; light impeccable, unmixed,
Made accurate the swallow's traveling print
Over the pasture, till he saw it fixed
Perfectly on a little patch of mint.
And he could feel in his body, driven home,
The wild tooth of the wolf that suckled Rome.

What if he came and stood beside my tree,
A poor, transparent thing with nothing to do,
His chest showing a jagged vacancy
Through which I might admire the distant view?
My house is solid, and the windows house
In their fine membranes the gelatinous light,
But darkness follows, and the dark allows
Obscure hints of a tapping sound at night.
And yet it may be merely that I dream
A woodpecker attacks the attic beam.

It is a well the light keeps him away;
We should have little to say in days like these,
Although once friends. We should have little to say,
But that there will be much planting of fig trees,
And Venus shall be clad in the prim leaf,
And turn a solitary. And her god, forgot,
Cast by that emblem out, shall spend his grief
Upon us. In that day the fruit shall rot

Unharvested. Then shall the sullen god
Perform his mindless fury in our blood.

Despair

Sadness. The moist gray shawls of drifting sea-fog,
Salting scrub pine, drenching the cranberry bogs,
Erasing all but foreground, making a ghost
Of anyone who walks softly away;
And the faint, penitent psalmody of the ocean.

Gloom. It appears among the winter mountains
On rainy days. Or the tiled walls of the subway
In caged and aging light, in the steel scream
And echoing vault of the departing train,
The vacant platform, the yellow destitute silence.

But despair is another matter. Midafternoon
Washes the worn bank of a dry arroyo,
Its ocher crevices, unrelieved rusts,
Where a startled lizard pauses, nervous, exposed
To the full glare of relentless marigold sunshine.

Richard Hugo

(1923–1982)

In Your War Dream

You must fly your 35 missions again.
The old base is reopened. The food is still bad.
You are disturbed. The phlegm you choked up
mornings in fear returns. You strangle on the phlegm.
You ask, "Why must I do this again?" A man
replies, "Home." You fly over one country
after another. The nations are bright like a map.
You pass over the red one. The orange one ahead
looks cold. The purple one north of that is the one
you must bomb. A wild land. Austere. The city
below seems ancient. You are on the ground.
Lovers are inside a cabin. You ask to come in.
They say "No. Keep watch on Stark Yellow Lake."
You stand beside the odd water. A terrible wind
keeps knocking you down. "I'm keeping watch
on the lake," you yell at the cabin. The lovers
don't answer. You break into the cabin. Inside
old women bake bread. They yell, "Return to the base."
You must fly your 35 missions again.

Cape Nothing

The sea designed these cliffs. Stone is cut
away odd places like a joke.
A suicide took aim, then flew out
in the arc he thought would find the sea.

He came down hearing "sucker" in the wind,
heard it break at "suck-" and all the time
tide was planning to ignore his bones.

Far out, the first white roll begins.
What an easy journey to this shore,
gliding miles of water over stars
and mudshark bones that laugh through tons
of green. You can time that wave and wind
by tripling your memory of oars.
The sea will con the gold from our remains.

Foam is white. When not, no dirtier
than bones gone brown with waiting for the sea.
When wind deposits spray on bone
bone begins to trickle down the sand.
Now the bones are gone, another shark
abandoned to the sea's refractive lie.
The moon takes credit for the boneless rock.

Bones don't really laugh beneath the sea.
They yawn and frown through green at time
and lie in squares to kid the moon
and drive stars from the water with the gleam
of phosphorus gone mad. Now a diver
poses on the cliff for passing cars
before he flies out singing "water, I am yours"

Letter to Logan from Milltown

Dear John: This a Dear John letter from booze.
With you, liver. With me, bleeding ulcer. The results
are the horrific same: as drunks we're done. Christ,
John, what a loss to those underground political
movements that count, the Degradationists,
the Dipsomaniacists, and that force gaining momentum

all over the world, the Deteriorationists. I hope
you know how sad this is. Once I quit drinking it was clear
to others, including our chairman (who incidentally
also had to quit drinking), that less 40 pounds
I look resolute and strong and on the surface appear
efficient. Try this for obscene development: they made me
director of creative writing. Better I'd gone on bleeding
getting whiter and whiter and finally blending
into the snow to be found next spring, a tragedy
that surely would increase my poetic reputation.
POET FOUND IN THAW   SNOWS CLAIM MISSOULA BARD
I'm in Milltown. You remember that bar, that beautiful bar
run by Harold Herndon where I pissed five years away
but pleasantly. And now I can't go in for fear
I'll fall sobbing to the floor. God, the ghosts in there.
The poems. Those honest people from the woods and mill.
What a relief that was from school, from that smelly
student-teacher crap and those dreary committees
where people actually say "considering the lateness
of the hour." Bad times too. That depressing summer
of '66 and that woman going—I've talked too often
about that. Now no bourbon to dissolve the tension,
to find self-love in blurred fantasies, to find the charm
to ask a woman home. What happens to us, John?
We are older than our scars. We have outlasted and survived
our wars and it turns out we're not as bad as we thought.
And that's really sad. But as a funny painter said
at a bash in Portland, and I thought of you then,
give Mother Cabrini another Martini. But not ever again
you and me. Piss on sobriety, and take care. Dick.

James Schuyler

(1923–1991)

The Payne Whitney Poems: What

What's in those pills?
After lunch and I can
hardly keep my eyes
open. Oh, for someone to
talk small talk with.
Even a dog would do.

Why are they hammering
iron outside? And what
is that generator whose
fierce hum comes in
the window? What is a
poem, anyway.

The daffodils, the heather
and the freesias all
speak to me. I speak
back, like St. Francis
and the wolf of Gubbio.

The Payne Whitney Poems: Pastime

I pick up a loaded pen and twiddle it.
After the blizzard
cold days of shrinking snow.
At visiting hours the cars
below my window form up

in a traffic jam. A fast-
moving man is in charge,
herding the big machines
like cattle. Weirdly, it all
keeps moving somehow. I read
a dumb detective story. I
clip my nails: they are as hard
as iron or glass. The clippers
keep sliding off them. Today
I'm shaky. A shave, a bath.
Chat. The morning paper.
Sitting. Staring. Thinking blankly.
TV. A desert kind of life.

The Payne Whitney Poems: The Night

The night is filled with indecisions
To take a downer or an upper
To take a walk
To lie
Down and relax

I order you: RELAX

To face the night
Alight—or dark—the air
Conditioner
The only song:
I love you so
Right now I need you so
So tired and so upset
And yet I mustn't phone:
I didn't know
I touched a wound that never healed
A trauma: wounds will heal
And all I did

Was panic so briefly
On the phone
"Oh baby! you scared me."
No, what you said
First on the phone
Was, "Baby I'll be right there."
You were. You did. You
Came, it seemed, as fast
As light, you love me so.
I didn't know someone
Once hurt you so,
Went suicidal: head in the oven
Threat—that
Hysteria bit. Not
My trip.
I am not suicidal:
We are strong and
You know it and
Yet
I must sleep
And wait—I
    love you so
You will know
I know you do
Already know:
We love each other
So. Good night
My own, my love
My dear, my dearest dear
It's true
We do we
Love each
Other so

Donald Justice

(1925–2004)

Counting the Mad

This one was put in a jacket,
This one was sent home,
This one was given bread and meat
But would eat none,
And this one cried No No No No
All day long.

This one looked at the window
As though it were a wall,
This one saw things that were not there,
This one things that were,
And this one cried No No No No
All day long.

This one thought himself a bird,
This one a dog,
And this one thought himself a man,
An ordinary man,
And cried and cried No No No No
All day long.

The Man Closing Up

1
Like a deserted beach,
The man closing up.

Broken glass on the rocks,
And seaweed coming in
To hang up on the rocks.

Old pilings, rotted, broken like teeth,
Where a pier was,

A mouth,
And the tide coming in.

The man closing up
Is like this.

2
He has no hunger
For anything,
The man closing up.

He would even try stones,
If they were offered.

But he has no hunger
For stones.

3
He would make his bed,
If he could sleep on it.

He would make his bed with white sheets
And disappear into the white,

Like a man diving,
If he could be certain

That the light
Would not keep him awake,

The light that reaches
To the bottom

4
The man closing up
Tries the doors.

But first
He closes the windows.

And before that even
He had looked out the windows.

There was no storm coming
That he could see.

There was no one out walking
At that hour.

Still,
He closes the windows
And tries the doors.

He knows about storms
And about people

And about hours
Like that one.

5
There is a word for it,
A simple word,
And the word goes around.

It curves like a staircase,
And it goes up like a staircase,
And it *is* a staircase,

An iron staircase
On the side of a lighthouse.
All in his head.

And it makes no sound at all
In his head,
Unless he says it.

Then the keeper
Steps on the rung,
The bottom rung,

And the ascent begins.
Clangorous,
Rung after rung.

He wants to keep the light going,
If he can.

But the man closing up
Does not say the word.

Allen Ginsberg

(1926–1997)

from "Howl"

I

I saw the best minds of my generation destroyed by madness,
   starving hysterical naked,

dragging themselves through the negro streets at dawn looking for
   an angry fix,

angelheaded hipsters burning for the ancient heavenly connection to
   the starry dynamo in the machinery of night,

who poverty and tatters and hollow-eyed and high sat up smoking in
   the supernatural darkness of cold-water flats floating across
   the tops of cities contemplating jazz,

who bared their brains to Heaven under the El and saw
   Mohammedan angels staggering on tenement roofs illuminated,

who passed through universities with radiant cool eyes hallucinating
   Arkansas and Blake-light tragedy among the scholars of war,

who were expelled from the academies for crazy & publishing
   obscene odes on the windows of the skull,

who cowered in unshaven rooms in underwear, burning their money
   in wastebaskets and listening to the Terror through the wall,

who got busted in their pubic beards returning through Laredo with
   a belt of marijuana for New York,

who ate fire in paint hotels or drank turpentine in Paradise Alley,
   death, or purgatoried their torsos night after night

with dreams, with drugs, with waking nightmares, alcohol and cock
and endless balls,

incomparable blind streets of shuddering cloud and lightning in the
mind leaping toward poles of Canada & Paterson, illuminating all
the moionless world of Time between,

Peyote solidities of halls, backyard green tree cemetery dawns,
wine drunkenness over the rooftops, storefront boroughs of
teahead joyride neon blinking traffic light, sun and moon and tree
vibrations in the roaring winter dusks of Brooklyn, ashcan rantings
and kind king light of mind,

who chained themselves to subways for the endless ride from Battery
to holy Bronx on benzedrine until the noise of wheels and children
brought them down shuddering mouth-wracked and battered
bleak of brain all drained of brilliance in the drear light of Zoo,

who sank all night in submarine light of Bickford's floated out and sat
through the stale beer afternoon in desolate Fugazzi's, listening to
the crack of doom on the hydrogen jukebox,

. . .

who studied Plotinus Poe St. John of the Cross telepathy and bop
kabbalah because the cosmos instinctively vibrated at their feet
in Kansas,

who loned it through the streets of Idaho seeking visionary indian
angels who were visionary indian angels,

who thought they were only mad when Baltimore gleamed in
supernatural ecstasy,

. . .

who demanded sanity trials accusing the radio of hypnotism & were
left with their insanity & their hands & a hung jury,

who threw potato salad at CCNY lecturers on Dadaism and
subsequently presented themselves on the granite steps of the
madhouse with shaven heads and harlequin speech of suicide,
demanding instantaneous lobotomy,

and who were given instead the concrete void of insulin Metrazol electricity hydrotherapy psychotherapy occupational therapy pingpong & amnesia,

who in humorless protest overturned only one symbolic pingpong table, resting briefly in catatonia,

returning years later truly bald except for a wig of blood, and tears and fingers, to the visible madman doom of the wards of the madtowns of the East,

Pilgrim State's Rockland's and Greystone's foetid halls, bickering with the echoes of the soul, rocking and rolling in the midnight solitude-bench dolmen-realms of love, dream of life a nightmare, bodies turned to stone as heavy as the moon . . .

. . .

Robert Bly

(1926–)

Depression

I felt my heart beat like an engine high in the air,
Like those scaffolding engines standing only on planks;
My body hung about me like an old grain elevator,
Useless, clogged, full of blackened wheat.
My body was sour, my life dishonest, and I fell asleep.

I dreamt that men came toward me, carrying thin wires;
I felt the wires pass in, like fire; they were old Tibetans,
Dressed in padded clothes, to keep out cold;
Then three work gloves, lying fingers to fingers,
In a circle, came toward me, and I awoke.

Now I want to go back among the dark roots;
Now I want to see the day pulling its long wing;
I want to see nothing more than two feet high;
I want to see no one, I want to say nothing,
I want to go down and rest in the black earth of silence.

Wiley Clements

(1928–)

Military Journalist

On the road outside Inchon,
in nondescript attire,
part G.I., part civilian,
less likely to draw fire,
heading for the line,

first horror that I saw:
a charbroiled North Korean
sprouting from the maw
of a rocket-shattered Russian
tank, T-thirty-four;
black flower in the sun,
the first of many more.

The next I came upon
I had not seen die.
There beside his gun,
a bullet through his eye,
a boy no older than
myself, his skull a flower,
petals of bone and skin.
A momentary shower
had washed the brain within
white as ivory:
I stared and then walked on;
he rose and walked with me.

Burned and shattered flowers,
young men who had no say,
dead soldiers, theirs and ours,
walk with me today.

Anne Sexton

(1928–1974)

from "The Double Image"

1.

I am thirty this November.
You are still small, in your fourth year.
We stand watching the yellow leaves go queer,
flapping in the winter rain,
falling flat and washed. And I remember
mostly the three autumns you did not live here.
They said I'd never get you back again.
I tell you what you'll never really know:
all the medical hypothesis
that explained my brain will never be as true as these
struck leaves letting go.

I, who chose two times
to kill myself, had said your nickname
the mewling months when you first came;
until a fever rattled
in your throat and I moved like a pantomime
above your head. Ugly angers spoke to me. The blame,
I heard them say, was mine. They tattled
like green witches in my head, letting doom
leak like a broken faucet;
as if doom had flooded my belly and filled your bassinet,
and old debt I must assume.

Death was simpler than I'd thought.
The day life made you well and whole
I let the witches take away my guilty soul.
I pretended I was dead
until the white men pumped the poison out,
putting me armless and washed through the rigamarole
of talking boxes and the electric bed.

I laughed to see the private iron in that hotel.
Today the yellow leaves
go queer. You ask me where they go. I say today believed
in itself, or else it fell.

Today, my small child, Joyce,
love your self's self where it lives.
There is no special God to refer to; or if there is,
why did I let you grow
in another place. You did not know my voice
when I came back to call. All the superlatives
of tomorrow's white tree and mistletoe
will not help you know the holidays you had to miss.
The time I did not love
myself, I visited your shoveled walks; you held my glove.
There was new snow after this.

. . .

The Addict

Sleepmonger,
deathmonger,
with capsules in my palms each night,
eight at a time from sweet pharmaceutical bottles
I make arrangements for a pint-sized journey.
I'm the queen of this condition.
I'm an expert on making the trip
and now they say I'm an addict.
Now they ask why.
Why!

Don't they know
that I promised to die!
I'm keeping in practice.
I'm merely staying in shape.

The pills are a mother, but better,
every color and as good as sour balls.
I'm on a diet from death.

Yes, I admit
it has gotten to be a bit of a habit—
blows eight at a time, socked in the eye,
hauled away by the pink, the orange,
the green and the white goodnights.
I'm becoming something of a chemical
mixture.
That's it!

My supply
of tablets
has got to last for years and years.
I like them more than I like me.
Stubborn as hell, they won't let go.
It's a kind of marriage.
It's a kind of war
where I plant bombs inside
of myself.

Yes
I try
to kill myself in small amounts,
an innocuous occupation.
Actually I'm hung up on it.
But remember I don't make too much noise.
And frankly no one has to lug me out
and I don't stand there in my winding sheet.
I'm a little buttercup in my yellow nightie
eating my eight loaves in a row
and in a certain order as in
the laying on of hands
or the black sacrament.

It's a ceremony
but like any other sport
it's full of rules.
It's like a musical tennis match where

my mouth keeps catching the ball.
Then I lie on my altar
elevated by the eight chemical kisses.

What a lay me down this is
with two pink, two orange,
two green, two white goodnights.
Fee-fi-fo-fum—
Now I'm borrowed.
Now I'm numb.

Ringing the Bells

And this is the way they ring
the bells in Bedlam
and this is the bell-lady
who comes each Tuesday morning
to give us a music lesson
and because the attendants make you go
and because we mind by instinct,
like bees caught in the wrong hive,
we are the circle of the crazy ladies
who sit in the lounge of the mental house
and smile at the smiling woman
who passes us each a bell,
who points at my hand
that holds my bell, E flat,
and this is the gray dress next to me
who grumbles as if it were special
to be old, to be old,
and this is the small hunched squirrel girl
on the other side of me
who picks at the hairs over her lip,
who picks at the hairs over her lip all day,
and this is how the bells really sound,

as untroubled and clean
as a workable kitchen,
and this is always my bell responding
to my hand that responds to the lady
who points at me, E flat;
and although we are no better for it,
they tell you to go. And you do.

Carl Wolfe Solomon

(1928–)

Anti-Totalitarian Manifesto for Evergreen Review

(after 5 years of imprisonment for yelling at my mother)

Every psychiatrist is a prick. Literature and psychiatry are incompatible. These people are sophists.
Conrad believes in evil; Freud doesn't. Freud is hor-
shit as Reich, his collaborator's imprisonment in Lewisburg proves. Sullivan was a paranoid. Do I have to
pay these European refugee birds and their American
competitors, the Sullivanians, to keep from being
put into a straitjacket, to keep from—Aw shit
they are keeping me in a bughouse accused of para-
noia because I refuse to pay the pettifogging
fucks. They are quacks. Admit it publicly. The
handmaiden of timid librarians—10 years of
these cocksuckers. Drop dead to every American
Psychoanalytic Review. They're just phonies. No
Ginsberg isn't mad.
Carl Solomon
And I'm not either. Long live infinity. Long
live Ginsberg. Viennese prurient bourgeois crap.
Friendly reader in your other-directed household,
The "Irrational Man" is your friend. Join me in my
fight for freedom. Down with every mush-mouthed auth-
or who pays lip-service to an unproven "Science" with a
paraphenalia of worthless medicines and contraptions
which cost lives—because it is stylish. It's stylish
because they have loot and the patients don't. It's the
new Gestapo. I never did nothing wrong. You read my article—so I like Isou and Artaud. Why the fuck am I
being held. I shit in your mouth. VIVE LAUTREAMONT. I'm
just a nice boy. Why don't you the American Public get
me out if it's such a nice country?

Ned O'Gorman

(1929–)

Peace, After Long Madness

After a long madness peace is an assassin
in the heart. Where there had been the clenched
fist, the strung out sinew, the hamstrung grin,
the erect eye and hand on every shadow like a spy,
now the river springs from the crystal of its sleep
in a sapphire lunge to the sea. A year of madness
is a libation poured out of nettles and boiled
herbs, of knives oiled with honey that cut silently
to the spine. I was madness's kin, no, more its
parent blood, its coursing lymph, its skeleton.
I kept company with lunacy, broke bread with him,
lay beside him, my head in his arms, felt him draw
down the sheet to watch me as I shook and so it was
one year till now.
Now the rocks become a sweetness
in the listless meadow, the lutist brays to
the ashes, flowers in the red crystal bowl push
against the windowpane and I sleep again,
my hands beneath my cheek, legs straight out,
eyes shut against the inward stratagem of dream
and the bedsheets and counterpane lie upon me
no more leaded capes of knobbed steel, but companions
of my skin, like the surface of my river is kindred
balm to the volcanoes and riven headlands that lie beneath it like pain.

Stuart Z. Perkoff

(1930–1974)

from "The Venice Poems, I"

4.
spring & summer
months of magic

>   from venice
>   to new york
>   a letter:

dear david/
>   monday, july 9, 1956
suzan
desperate after
weeks of struggle with
what was a terrifying combination of

>   numinous
>   paranoid
>   insightful

>   pressures

& pressures

entered,with a glad relief
&,
>   (on my part also
prayer

the general hospital
psychiatric unit

where she is now
where i go to see her again today
where all my hope & agony are now entombed

there are explanations, as you must know
impossible
to make

a loss
            (if what is lost is, precisely
                    everything
                    that is /
                        reality

is too much more than just the word
to investigate fully

            i was observer
            & involved participant
            in all aspects of it

what i wd like now
to recreate, is that role:
the onlooker of love.

but i cannot put down a chronology
of the events.

a beginning is a growing thing. "people"
says Olson, somewhere in the wild *maximus*
"dont change. they only stand/more revealed."

possibly certain things in letters
over the past month
indicated happenings.

possibly certain things in letters
over the past years
indicated happenings.

possibly certain things in lives
over the past centuries
indicated happenings.

            inflated with the Divine Mother
reliving traumas of her births

      searching the wild beds & hatreds of the world
for her twin

      her strength
her unhad power

      david, david
the tears that flowed!
that there cd be such tears!

      there were too many things for her to see
      she cd not sort them out

into herself, & me, the world & time
      into space & history
         she sent her eyes & vision

the warps & stones & enveloping structures
      she saw thru
        or around

until she came to that point in her mind
      where they were of enormous size
        & shapes completely without reference

& she sd: "hit me, feed me, rape me, touch me
      do something real to me, that I may know, touch, have
        something real to hold to. i
          must have something to
          hold to."

there is only so much that can be accomplished
by love.
beginnings are growing things.
there came a boundary, & i against it
stunned all my sharpness.

there came that boundary
& i, exhausted
      had nothing more to give
& only saw insanity in her eyes
& in my own.

              beyond that time
i can as yet record little.
on the level of simple fact
i can say
that she entered the hospital of her own desire
& has so strongly a need to be helped

              (by them, her lifetime enemies, the doctors
                  their white coats terrifying her dreams
                  since childhood

that i accept it
& am aware that it is good
that she is there

but the tears, that have flowed.
david
david
that there cd be

such tears.

o burning eyes on the post office wall
o citybuilder, moneymaker, oilwell & fun-zone
at the playground at the foot of yr city
the women drive each other mad
their children hang limp & screaming from the pleasure machines

o builder of canals & real estate profits
touched by eyes
at the sea
things happen

              the fog
              the lites
              the people & stores

Junk Nursery Rhymes

1.

mother, may i go out to fix?
yes, my darling daughter
you may tie yr arm & punch yr vein
but fill the spike with water

2.

sing a sick a song dance
arm full of cry
20 grains of morphine
shot into yr eye
when the eye is open
the world beings to sing, & sting
so fix my lads, & lassies, too
for crying is the thing

3.

sick jack horner
stood on the corner
waiting to meet with the man
he stood thru the nite
& into the lite
for all i know there he still stands

poor jack

4.

o do you know the hungry monk?
the hungry monk?
the hungry monk?
o do you know the hungry monk, he lives
between yr shoulders

yes i know the hungry monk
the hungry monk
the hungry monk
yes i know the hungry monk
he lives between my shoulders

5.

junkie, junkie, where have you been?
trying to score, out in the scene.
junkie, junkie, did you score enuf?
if there was that much, it wdn't be stuff.

6.

to market, to market to cop half a gram
into my arm to find the spike jammed

all over town to borrow a gun
fixed under a street lite / o had lots of fun

risk & adventure / run out of breath
my special market sells wings of death

7.

there was a young poet who lived in a zoo
he listened / he was human
he did what he cd do

he hated the murder of his legs & arms
he insulted the monkey
so it brought him harm
it put him in jail / now he dreams of his need
while the monk runs the streets on a new hungry steed

8.

bleeding rotten
he stole the cotton
hoping he wd fly

he got busted for those marks
& wasnt even high

Sylvia Plath

(1932–1963)

Elm

I know the bottom, she says. I know it with my great tap root:
It is what you fear.
I do not fear it: I have been there.

Is it the sea you hear in me,
Its dissatisfactions?
Or the voice of nothing, that was your madness?

Love is a shadow.
How you lie and cry after it
Listen: these are its hooves: it has gone off, like a horse.

All night I shall gallop thus, impetuously,
Till your head is a stone, your pillow a little turf,
Echoing, echoing.

Or shall I bring you the sound of poisons?
This is rain now, this big hush.
And this is the fruit of it: tin-white, like arsenic.

I have suffered the atrocity of sunsets.
Scorched to the root
My red filaments burn and stand, a hand of wires.

Now I break up in pieces that fly about like clubs.
A wind of such violence
Will tolerate no bystanding: I must shriek.

The moon, also, is merciless: she would drag me
Cruelly, being barren.
Her radiance scathes me. Or perhaps I have caught her.

I let her go. I let her go
Diminished and flat, as after radical surgery.
How your bad dreams possess and endow me.

I am inhabited by a cry.
Nightly it flaps out
Looking, with its hooks, for something to love.

I am terrified by this dark thing
That sleeps in me;
All day I feel its soft, feathery turnings, its malignity.

Clouds pass and disperse.
Are those the faces of love, those pale irretrievables?
Is it for such I agitate my heart?

I am incapable of more knowledge.
What is this, this face
So murderous in its strangle of branches?———

Its snaky acids hiss
It petrifies the will. These are the isolate, slow faults
That kill, that kill, that kill.

Street Song

By a mad miracle I go intact
Among the common rout
Thronging sidewalk, street,
And bickering shops;
Nobody blinks a lid, gapes,
Or cries that this raw flesh
Reeks of the butcher's cleaver,
Its heart and guts hung hooked
And bloodied as a cow's split frame
Parceled out by white-jacketed assassins.

Oh no, for I strut it clever
As a greenly escaped idiot,
Buying wine, bread,
Yellow-casqued chrysanthemums—
Arming myself with the most reasonable items
To ward off, at all cost, suspicions
Roused by thorned hands, feet, head,
And that great wound
Squandering red
From the flayed side.

Even as my each mangled nerve-end
Trills its hurt out
Above pitch of pedestrian ear,
So, perhaps I, knelled dumb by your absence,
Alone can hear
Sun's parched scream,
Every downfall and crash
Of gutted star,
And, more daft than any goose,
This cracked world's incessant gabble and hiss.

from *The Journal of Saint Dympna*

(Earl "Pete" Nurmi, editor)
(published 1979)

Lee Merrill
Medication

I took a white cogentin
And a yellow thorazine
I took a demi-dixie-cup
Of water in between.

I took a white cogentin
And a yellow thorazine,
I think they tried to help us keep
From the things we'd seen.

Medication, medication, medication—
It is so good for you,
It is so good for the nation.
No more sadness
And no more elation!
Medication, medication, medication.

I took a white cogentin
And a yellow thorazine,
I took a demi-dixie-cup
Of water in between,
I knew Napoleon of France
I knew sweet Joan of Arc,
I knew a man who walked his dog,
But it would not bark.

Medication, medication, medication—
So good for you,
So good for the nation.
There will be no more sadness

And no more elation:
Medication, medication, medication.

I took a white cogentin
And a yellow thorazine,
I took a demi-dixie-cup
Of water in between:

I took a walk with the man
And what he talked about
Was that if I'd be a good boy
He would let me out.

from *The Journal of Saint Dympna*

(Earl "Pete" Nurmi, editor)
(published 1979)

Mary Coleman
"The ghost behemians of Meridel LeSueur"

The ghost behemians of Meridel LeSueur
people the shadows of Loring park.
We throw old crackers across thin ice.
Then skate the fat ducks toward food.
One orange web slips, recovers, slips
recovers, slips forward. /Here come
waddling more fat ducks, skating.
All the ducks come, green heads flashing
in the sun./ And from the blue air seagulls/
weave and dive./My thighs polymorphously
ripple:/as if, Leda like, gods incarnate/
dive for me./ The December click-cold air
benches are empty/and none wanders or waits/
only Meridel's ghost behemians through
frost incarnations, in the trees laughing.

from *The Journal of Saint Dympna*

(Earl "Pete" Nurmi, editor)
(published 1979)

John Appling Sours
Institute at Christmas

Going back to the cold wind crossing
      the Hudson River/
and sweeping Washington Heights

I see glass that gives back gold to
      the east/
and cast their radiance on faces
pressed against dirty windows crossed
      by bars/

The terrace is blown free of chairs
      and umbrellas
where last summer's patients played
      checkers/
or look down on cars in a caravan

and tomorrow they will come to rounds and
take their place in the circle with social
      workers/
they will ask for discharges but only light
      will shine/
across the floor
framing those objects whose spirit is
bathed in lithium ions

While in the common room lie yellowed
      cotton clumps/
pierced by needles brittle from thirst.
A woman files her nails in unspeakable silence
and on the childrens ward

a little girl bangs her head against
the green walls

and several floors away
psychiatrists sip eggnog in the lounge
they talk about Freud and Jung, or
Descartes and Sartre, and stuff
their meerschaums full of cavendish.

Lucille Clifton

(1936–)

shapeshifter poems

1

the legend is whispered
in the women's tent
how the moon when she rises
full
follows some men into themselves
and changes them there
the season is short
but dreadful   shapeshifters
they wear strange hands
they walk through the houses
at night   their daughters
do not know them

2

who is there to protect her
from the hands of the father
not the windows which see and
say nothing   not the moon
that awful eye   not the woman
she will become with her
scarred tongue   who   who   who   the owl
laments into the evening who
will protect her   this   prettylittlegirl

3

if the little girl lies
still enough
shut enough
hard enough
shapeshifter may not
walk tonight

the full moon may not
find him here
the hair on him
bristling
rising
up

    4
the poem at the end of the world
is the poem the little girl breathes
into her pillow   the one
she cannot tell   the one
there is no one to hear   this poem
is a political poem   is a war poem   is a
universal poem but is not about
these things   this poem
is about one human heart this   poem
is the poem at the end of the world

Jim Harrison

(1937–)

Noon

Spring: despondency,
fall: despair,
onset of winter
a light rain in the heart
the pony tethered to the telephone
pole day after day until he's eaten
the circle, moved to another pole,
another circle: winter never deepens
but falls dead upon the ground,
body of the sky whirled
in gray gusts:
from Manitoba stretched brains
of north; heat for heart, head,
in smallest things—dry socks,
strange breasts, an ounce of sun
glittering above the blue shadows
of the barn.

Sequence I

The mad have black roots in their brains
around which vessels clot and embrace
each other as mating snakes.

The roots feed on the brain until the brain
is all root—now the brain is gray
and suffocates in its own folds.

287

The brain grows smaller and beats
against its cage of bone
like a small wet bird.

Let us pity the mad we see every day,
the bird is dying without air and water
and growing smaller,
the air is cold, her beak is sharp,
the beating shriller.

Les Murray

(1938–)

from *Fredy Neptune*, Book I

. . .

Now Turkey was in, and Russia's last trade lifeline blocked
so she would rot. It was all we'd come to do, I worked out later.
We idled and dressed ship round the City and Black Sea
playing skat, eating goulash.
When Gallipoli came, I thought: I will desert
if I have to fight Australians. But instead
my mates and I, on shore leave up by Trabzon
at last saw women with their faces unwrapped in the open.

They were huddling, terrified, crying.
crossing themselves, in the middle of men all yelling.
Their big loose dresses were sopping. Kerosene, you could smell it.
The men were prancing, feeling them, poking at them to dance—
then pouf! they were alight, the women, dark wicks to great
   orange flames,
whopping and shrieking. If we'd had rifles there
we'd have massacred those bastards. We had only fists and boots.
One woman did cuddle a man: he went up screaming too.

. . .

The first time I slipped up badly was on that voyage.
We had a deck galley. The cook, a different cook, he was a drunk
and the fire had been doused, in dirty weather. The boy was
   relighting it
with kerosene, and it blew out and caught his clothes.
He was screaming blind when I reached him, half the galley
   alight too
and when I got him put out I didn't notice
I had caught, here, all up my calf, you can see it.
They took the boy out, and there I'm tidying up, still burning.

The cook started screaming, I didn't know what at.
One of his blue dragons had come real. I went on burning—
see how deep it goes in? The little silver walls?
The supercargo whopped me out with a soaking jumper
and everybody near was looking. *He devil!* screams the cook
he walk in fire, not hurt. You stay away, you devil!—
You'd know, I said. But the word I was uncanny made the skipper
get rid of me. Or I might have had a midnight flotation test.

There was no pain in the leg, not burning, not healing. It stank
and I used a farm cure on that: metho, poured on neat and smoky.
By the time it healed up, much as it ever would, I'd lost
my leprosy-thinking. I was young again, becalmed in port, curious,
scratching up dust a bit. A café waitress there noticed
and helped me out. This part is awful to admit.
She had to tell me everything. *Oh yes, you're ready, yes,*
and *Stop, hey, you're finished. I'm flooded. Didn't you feel that?*

· · ·

Sharon Olds

(1942–)

Satan Says

I am locked in a little cedar box
with a picture of shepherds pasted onto
the central panel between carvings.
The box stands on curved legs.
It has a gold, heart-shaped lock
and no key. I am trying to write my
way out of the closed box
redolent of cedar. Satan
comes to me in the locked box
and says, *I'll get you out. Say*
My father is a shit. I say
my father is a shit and Satan
laughs and says, *It's opening.*
Say your mother is a pimp.
My mother is a pimp. Something
opens and breaks when I say that.
My spine uncurls in the cedar box
like the pink back of the ballerina pin
with a ruby eye, resting beside me on
satin in the cedar box.
Say shit, say death, say fuck the father,
Satan says, down my ear.
The pain of the locked past buzzes
in the child's box on her bureau, under
the terrible round pond eye
etched around with roses, where
self-loathing gazed at sorrow.
Shit. Death. Fuck the father.
Something opens. Satan says
Don't you feel a lot better?
Light seems to break on the delicate
edelweiss pin, carved in two

colors of wood. I love him too,
you know, I say to Satan dark
in the locked box. I love them but
I'm trying to say what happened to us
in the lost past. *Of course*, he says
and smiles, *of course. Now say: torture.*
I see, through blackness soaked in cedar,
the edge of a large hinge open.
Say: the father's cock, the mother's
cunt, says Satan, *I'll get you out.*
The angle of the hinge widens
until I see the outlines of
the time before I was, when they were
locked in the bed. When I say
the magic words, Cock, Cunt,
Satan softly says, *Come out.*
But the air around the opening
is heavy and thick as hot smoke.
Come in, he says, and I feel his voice
breathing from the opening.
The exit is through Satan's mouth.
Come in my mouth, he says, *you're there*
already, and the huge hinge
begins to close. Oh no, I loved
them, too, I brace
my body tight
in the cedar house.
Satan sucks himself out the keyhole.
I'm left locked in the box, he seals
the heart-shaped lock with the wax of his tongue.
It's your coffin now, Satan says.
I hardly hear;
I am warming my cold
hands at the dancer's
ruby eye—
the fire, the suddenly discovered knowledge of love.

Timothy Dekin

(1943–2001)

Melancholy

Morning, old promise of relief,
Asserts its presence with a light
Unsympathetic, and too bright,
And you are easier with grief,

The amber glowing through drawn shades.
You sit and smoke. Through muted fire
The dust shifts only to expire
On quilt or rug. The bed's unmade,

There's nothing to be gained, or known,
Or saved. Tomorrow you'll be stronger.
Rest here in peace a little longer.
Some cannot make it on their own.

Quincy Troupe

(1943–)

River Town Packin House Blues

Big Tom was a black nigguh man,
cold & black,
eye say Big Tom was a black nigguh man,
black steel flesh,
standin like a gladiator, soaked in
animal blood, bits of flesh,
wringin wet,
standin at the center of death,
buzzards hoverin, swingin his hammer called death,
260 workdays,
swingin his hammer named death

Big Tom was a black packin houseman,
thirty years,
eye say Big Tom was a black packin houseman,
loved them years,
& swang his hammer like ol John Henry
poundin nails.
swang that hammer twenty years
crushin skulls
of cows & pigs screamin fear
the man underneath slit their throats,
twenty years,
the man underneath slit their throats

Big Tom was a 'prentice for ten long years,
watchin death,
eye say Big Tom was 'prentice for ten long years,
smellin death,
was helper to a fat white man,
who got slow,
was helper to a fat white man,

who swang a hammer
till he couldnt do it no mo,
so he taught Big Tom how to kill
with a hammer,
he taught Big Tom how to kill

& twenty years of killin
is a lot to bring home,
eye say twenty years of killin
is a lot to bring home
& drinkin too much gin & whisky
can make a gentle/man blow
dont chu know
eye say drinkin too much
gin & whiskey
can make a good man
sho nuff blow,
dont chu know

Big Tom beat his wife after killin all day,
his six chillun too,
eye say Tom beat his wife after killin all day
his young chillun too,
beat em so awful bad, he beat em right out dey shoes,
screamin blues,
eye say he beat em so awful bad
he made a redeyed hungry alley rat spread the news
'bout dues
these black/blues people was payin, couldnt even bite em,
cause of the dues
these black/blues people was payin

Big Tom killed six men, maimed a couple a hundred
& never served a day,
eye say Big Tom killed six men, maimed a couple a
hundred,
never in jail one day,
the figures coulda been higher, but the smart ones,
they ran away,
eye say the number that was maimed, or dead, coulda
been higher,

but the smart ones,
they ran away, swallowin pride, saved from the graveyard,
another day,
the smart ones,
they ran away

Big Tom, workin all day, thirty years,
uh huh, sweatin heavy
Big Tom swingin his hamma, all right, twenty summers
outta love
Big Tom killin for pay,
Uh huh, twenty autumns, outta need,
Big Tom dealin out murders, like a houseman, all night,
in the painyards, outta false pride,
Big Tom drinkin heavy, uh huh,
laughin loose in taverns,
Big Tom loose
In Black communities, death fights cancels light,
& Big Tom keeps on, stumbling

& twenty years of killin
is too much to bring home to love,
eye say twenty years of killin
is too much to bring home to love,
& drinkin heavy gin & whiskey
can make a strong man fall in mud,
eye say drinkin too much/ gin & whiskey
can make a good man have bad blood
dont chu know
can make a strong
man have
bad blood

Big Black Tom was a cold nigguh man,
strong & black,
eye say Big Black Tom was a cold nigguh man,
hard steel flesh,
& stood like a gladiator, soaked in blood,
bits of flesh,
soakin wet,
stood at the center, in the middle of death,

sweatin vultures,
swingin his hamma called death, 260 workdays,
twenty years,
like ol John Henry,
eye say swingin his hammer named death

Thomas P. Beresford

(1946–)

Edith in Ann Arbor

"Where will it end?" she asked me one time, years ago,
Before it ended there and began somewhere else.
Indecency was an abstraction to be borne,
Not fought with. She was older, more adept
At life than I, and watching her was watching
Changelessness in the lunar face through dark and light.
Until one night the swinging corpse of a child in a closet
Woke me and the floating corpse of the same still child
Woke me again, killing the last indecency.
She bore it to an end. I fought it to a draw.
An ending and an endlessness was all we saw.

R. L. Barth

(1947–)

Epigraph from **Deeply Dug In**

I swore I'd only be a three year cypher
But learn each sweaty midnight I'm a lifer.

Jane Kenyon

(1947–1995)

Having it Out with Melancholy

1. FROM THE NURSERY

When I was born, you waited
behind a pile of linen in the nursery,
and when we were alone, you lay down
on top of me, pressing
the bile of desolation into every pore.

And from that day on
everything under the sun and moon
made me sad—even the yellow
wooden beads that slid and spun
along a spindle on my crib.

You taught me to exist without gratitude.
You ruined my manners toward God:
"We're here simply to wait for death;
the pleasures of earth are overrated."

I only appeared to belong to my mother,
to live among blocks and cotton undershirts
with snaps; among red tin lunch boxes
and report cards in ugly brown slipcases.
I was already yours—the anti-urge,
the mutilator of souls.

2. BOTTLES

Elavil, Ludiomil, Doxepin,
Norpramin, Prozac, Lithium, Xanax,
Wellbutrin, Parnate, Nardil, Zoloft.
The coated ones smell sweet or have
no smell; the powdery ones smell
like the chemistry lab at school
that made me hold my breath.

3. SUGGESTION FROM A FRIEND
You wouldn't be so depressed
if you really believed in God.

4. OFTEN
Often I go to bed as soon after dinner
as seems adult
(I mean I try to wait for dark)
in order to push away
from the massive pain in sleep's
frail wicker coracle.

5. ONCE THERE WAS LIGHT
Once, in my early thirties, I saw
that I was a speck of light in the great
river of light that undulates through time.

I was floating with the whole
human family. We were all colors—those
who are living now, those who have died,
those who are not yet born. For a few

moments I floated, completely calm,
and I no longer hated having to exist.

Like a crow who smells hot blood
you came flying to pull me out
of the glowing stream.
"I'll hold you up. I never let my dear
ones drown!" After that, I wept for days.

6. IN AND OUT
The dog searches until he finds me
upstairs, lies down with a clatter
of elbows, puts his head on my foot.

Sometimes the sound of his breathing
saves my life—in and out, in
and out; a pause, a long sigh. . . .

7. PARDON

A piece of burned meat
wears my clothes, speaks
in my voice, dispatches obligations
haltingly, or not at all.
It is tired of trying
to be stouthearted, tired
beyond measure.

We move on to the monoamine
oxidase inhibitors. Day and night
I feel as if I had drunk six cups
of coffee, but the pain stops
abruptly. With the wonder
and bitterness of someone pardoned
for a crime she did not commit
I come back to marriage and friends,
to pink fringed hollyhocks; come back
to my desk, books, and chair.

8. CREDO

Pharmaceutical wonders are at work
but I believe only in this moment
of well-being. Unholy ghost,
you are certain to come again.

Coarse, mean, you'll put your feet
on the coffee table, lean back,
and turn me into someone who can't
take the trouble to speak; someone
who can't sleep, or who does nothing
but sleep; can't read, or call
for an appointment for help.

There is nothing I can do
against your coming.
When I awake, I am still with thee.

9. WOOD THRUSH

High on Nardil and June light
I wake at four,

waiting greedily for the first
note of the wood thrush. Easeful air
presses through the screen
with the wild, complex song
of the bird, and I am overcome

by ordinary contentment.
What hurt me so terribly
all my life until this moment?
How I love the small, swiftly
beating heart of the bird
singing in the great maples;
its bright, unequivocal eye.

Yusef Komunyakaa

(1947–)

Losses

After Nam he lost himself,
   not trusting his hands
      with loved ones.

His girlfriend left,
   & now he scouts the edge of town,
      always with one ear

cocked & ready to retreat,
   to blend with hills, poised
      like a slipknot

becoming a noose.
   Unlike punji stakes,
      his traps only snag the heart.

Sometimes he turns in a circle
   until a few faces from Dak To
      track him down.

A dress or scarf in the distance
   can nail him to a dogwood.
      Down below, to his left,

from where the smog rises,
   a small voice reaches his ear
      somehow. No, never mind—

he's halfway back, closer to a ravine,
   going deeper into saw vines,
      in behind White Cove,

following his mind like a dark lover,
   away from car horns & backfire
      where only days are stolen.

Joseph Salemi

(1948–)

Sicilian Beachhead

He had to kill her, though it was not planned—
He crawled up that warm beach at night, in war.
Who could foresee a young girl on the sand,
A bicyclist along the moonlit shore?

She saw him. If he let the girl go free
She might raise an alarm. He was afraid.
The blued-steel bayonet came out, and he
Stabbed deep and hard, the full length of its blade.

Years later, troubled by a nagging ghost
Of doubt, he'd tell himself there was no blame.
If she had been a sentry at a post
No question that he would have done the same.

But every night he felt her fragile breath—
He languished, pined, and drank himself to death.

Aimee Grunberger

(1951–1995)

The Administration of Veterans

I just saw him, had to slow way down to be sure.
Whatever the opposite of remission is, this was it.
He stood there, an urban Robinson Crusoe,
sunburnt, barefoot, shirt in tatters, hair and beard electrified,
drinking the dregs of coffee cups at a sidewalk café.
Jabbing a finger in the air, giving the finger to City Hall
to the bank that calls itself Citizens'
to the boarded-up Union Station,
stranded on a trackless railbed.
He was keening in almost-Gaelic.
It might have been the wake of Parnell.

I remember how he once inspired the other vets.
So clean and sober in a borrowed jacket and tie,
prim as a bondbroker and full of jittery pride.
As long as Haldol kept the neural juices
from scorching his brain like lye,
he remained my prize patient. My success story.
Before he took off, signed himself out
as the shifts were changing,
he slipped this message under my office door:

Dogs no longer bark at me.
In my handbook, this state
is referred to as bliss.
But my time here is short.
I'm aging faster now, burning
up along the primitive circuitry.
Already older than
my mother and father put together,
and with so much
work left for me to do.

One more revolution in Kennedy Plaza.
Now that the light is red and everything has stopped,
his words come into audible focus.
Those pigs those fucking pigs they leave you with nothing.
He begins to cross.
Then the light goes mercifully green and I gun it.

Jimmy Santiago Baca

(1952–)

This Dark Side

has always haunted me,
fiercely adamant in its opposition
to all the good I create:
subversive and defiant.
While my spirit revels in light,
it
gorges on cesspool pleasures
leaving my spirit at times a fly
and maggot-infested carcass, dissembling
my dreamwork, disintegrating it back to sand
wind scatters, blows
back into my face
I have to lower in shame.

Imagine a ladder of light, a trellis of branches
rising out of my soul in blossoming radiance,
carving its own latticed speech in the sky
toward the sun.
Imagine
my dark side freeing the termites to gnaw
down these branches.
My soul
falls like a black oak tree cracked by an ice storm.
It stares up with a skull's nightmare grimace
of cruel suffering on its frozen face.
But hovering at dawn,
hope like a butterfly floats around it,
a powdery rainbow dust effusing the air
with pervasive peace.
And then
the morning yawns forth like whispering lilac
on the air.

My heart untangles itself from its dreams
like wild honeysuckle grandly striding into halls of sunlight,
trickling with dew beads of grace
that sigh from my lips.
Some power moves in me,
a divine dancer elegantly celebrating its existence.

I tell you now,
the dark side arrives unannounced
with cold hands,
scoffing at my efforts to live a single day in dignity,
undermining the goodness in me,
though I'm getting better at exposing it,
standing before it like a brittle twig
smashed under its wrecking tank tread.

All that I've despised and spat at in disgust
I've become at certain moments in life,
but I continue to praise the spirit,
refuse to embrace the utter horror
of self-destructive impulses.

I draw the curtains of my life shut,
a silent stranger to myself
chewing on the maddening, shredded remnants of my heart.
Accepting it as part of me, loving it,
not afraid of feeling its pain, understanding
how I always contradict myself,
I succumb to passion,
even indifference,
roar my loss and abandonment,
bell-bellow my cathedral soul,
trust and suspect
in a constant flight between light and dark.

It never ends. This harsh beauty,
this struggle not to retreat in fear
but to celebrate what's hard earned, staying true to myself,
is what it's all about.

Mark Jarman

(1952–)

Questions for Ecclesiastes

What if on a foggy night in a beachtown, a night when
    the Pacific leans close like the face of a wet cliff, a
    preacher were called to the house of a suicide, a
    house of strangers, where a child had discharged a
    rifle through the roof of her mouth and the top of
    her skull?

What if he went to the house where the parents, stunned
    into plaster statues, sat behind their coffee table,
    and what if he assured them that the sun would rise
    and go down, the wind blow south, then turn north,
    whirling constantly, rivers—even the concrete flume
    of the great Los Angeles—run into the sea, and four-
    teen year old girls would manage to spirit themselves
    out of life, nothing was new under the sun?

What if he said the eye is not satisfied with seeing, nor the
    ear filled with hearing? Would he want to view the
    bedroom vandalized by self-murder or hear the
    quiet before the tremendous shout of the gun or the
    people inside the shout, shouting or screaming,
    crying and pounding to get into the room, kicking
    through the hollow-core door and making a new
    sound and becoming a new silence—the silence he
    entered with his comfort?

What if as comfort he said to the survivors I praise the
    dead which are dead already more than the living,
    and better is he than both dead and living who is
    not yet alive? What if he folded his hands together
    and ate his own flesh in prayer? For he did pray
    with them. He asked them, the mother and father, if

they wished to pray to do so in any way they felt
comfortable, and the father knelt at the coffee table
and the mother turned to squeeze her eyes into a
corner of the couch, and they prayed by first listening to his prayer, then clawing at his measured
cadences with tears (the man cried) and curses (the
woman swore). What if, then, the preacher said be
not rash with thy mouth and let not thine heart be
hasty to utter anything before God: for God is in
heaven?

What if the parents collected themselves, then, and asked
him to follow them to their daughter's room, and
stood at the shattered door, the darkness of the
room beyond, and the father reached in to put his
hand on the light switch and asked if the comforter,
the preacher they were meeting for the first time in
their lives, would like to see the aftermath, and
instead of recoiling and apologizing, he said that
the dead know not anything for the memory of
them is forgotten? And while standing in the hall-
way, he noticed the shag carpet underfoot, like the
fur of a cartoon animal, the sort that requires comb-
ing with a plastic rake, leading into the bedroom,
where it would have to be taken up, skinned off the
concrete slab of the floor, and still he said for their
love and hatred and envy are now perished, neither
have the dead any more portion for ever in anything
that is done under the sun?

What if as an act of mercy so acute it pierced the preacher's
skull and traveled the length of his spine, the man
did not make him regard the memory of his daughter as it must have filled her room, but guided the
wise man, the comforter, to the front door, with his
wife with her arms crossed before her in that gesture we use to show a stranger to the door, acting
out a rite of closure, compelled to be social, as we
try to extricate ourselves by breaking off the exten-
sions of our bodies, as raccoons gnaw their legs from
traps, turning aside our gaze, letting only the numb

tissue of valedictory speech ease us apart, and the
preacher said live joyfully all the days of the life of
thy vanity, for that is thy portion in this life?

They all seem worse than heartless, don't they, these stark
and irrelevant platitudes, albeit stoical and final,
oracular, stony, and comfortless? But they were at
the center of that night, even if they were unspoken.

And what if one with only a casual connection to the
tragedy remembers a man, younger than I am today,
going out after dinner and returning, then sitting in
the living room, drinking a cup of tea, slowly
finding the strength to say he had visited these
grieving strangers and spent some time with them?

Still that night exists for people I do not know in ways I do
not know, though I have tried to imagine them. I
remember my father going out and my father coming back. The fog, like the underskin of a broken
wave, made a low ceiling that the street lights
pierced and illuminated. And God who shall bring
every work into judgement, with every secret thing,
whether it be good or whether it be evil, who could
have shared what he knew with people who needed
urgently to hear it, God kept a secret.

from "Transfiguration"

. . .

When we brought our mother to him, we said, "Lord,
she falls down the stairs.
She cannot hold her water. In the afternoon she forgets
the morning."
And he said, "All things are possible to those who believe.
Shave her head,

Insert a silicone tube inside her skull, and run it under
   her scalp,
Down her neck, and over her collarbone, and lead it into
   her stomach."
And we did and saw that she no longer stumbled or wet
   herself.
She could remember the morning until the evening came.
   And we went our way,
Rejoicing as much as we could, for we had worried many
   years.

. . .

Franz Wright

(1953–)

Voice

I woke up at 4 in the afternoon. Rain woke
me. Dark. Mail—a voice said, You'll have
mail,

scaring and gladdening my heart. Enough anyway
to get me out of bed, attempt to make coffee,
dress and begin limping down stairs. All

the boxes were empty. Of course. A voice said,
He just hasn't come yet. But I knew. It is 4
in the afternoon—the others have already taken

the mail indoors. Hours ago. If this my box
is empty now then it was always empty.

Rain. Darker

now. By the time I had walked, more or less,
back up the stairs, the treacherous voice had
nothing more to say.

Hope. They call it hope—

that obscene cruelty, it never lets up for a
minute.

But not anymore—never again. If the telephone
rings just don't answer, said the voice. Very
adaptable, the obsequious voice. If the mail does
come put it in the garbage with its fellow trash;
or set it on fire in that big metal can in the alley,
you know, your publisher. Dark. Odd. It was
light when I finally slept, I say out loud. I suppose I am insane now,

on top of everything else. He talks to himself now,
they'll say. Who. By the time you get back to your
room you won't even exist. A bit mean now. And you
will sit down in the chair with your back to the
window, it says.

After a while I know for a fact you will open your
notebook and write all this down,

why I don't know. No doubt you will even show it to
somebody, at some point: they'll talk to you, offer advice,

admit admiration for this phrase,

dislike for that. But they don't understand. You don't

care now—how can you. No, I don't care what they say,
what they do to me now. I used to. Terribly. And then you didn't.

And then I didn't.

Rorschach Test

To tell you the truth I'd have thought it had gone
out of use long ago; there is something so 19th Century
about it,

with its absurd reverse Puritanism.

Can withdrawal from reality or interpersonal inhibition
be gauged by uneasiness at being summoned to a small
closed room to discuss ambiguously sexual pictures with
a total stranger?

Alone in the presence of the grave examiner, it soon
becomes clear that, short of strangling yourself, you're

going to have to find a way of suppressing the snickers of
an eight year old sex fiend, and feign curiosity about
the process to mask your indignation at being placed in
this ridiculous situation.

Sure, you see lots of pretty butterflies with the faces of
ancient Egyptian queens, and so forth—you see other things,
too.

Flying stingray vaginas all over the place, along with a
few of their male counterparts transparently camouflaged
as who knows what pillars and swords out of the old brain's
unconscious.

You keep finding yourself thinking, "God damn it, don't tell
me that isn't a pussy!"

But after long silence come out with, "Oh, this must be
Christ trying to prevent a large crowd from stoning a
woman to death."

The thing to do is keep a straight face, which is hard. After
all, you're *supposed* to be crazy (and are probably proving it).

Maybe a nudge and a chuckle or two wouldn't hurt your
case. Yes,

it's some little card game you've gotten yourself into
this time, when your only chance is to lose. Fold,

and they have got you by the balls—

just like the ones you neglected to identify.

Certain Tall Buildings

I know a little
about it: I know
if you contemplate suicide
long enough, it
begins to contemplate you—
oh, it has plans for you.
It calls to your attention

the windows of certain tall
buildings, wooded snow fields
in your memory where you might cunningly vanish
to remotely, undiscoverably
sleep. Remember your mother
hanging the cat
in front of you when you were four?

Why not that? That
should fix her. Or deep drugs
glibly prescribed by psychiatrists weary
as you of your failure to change
into someone else—
you'll show them
change.

These thoughts, occuring once too often,
are no longer your own. No,
they think you.
The thing is not to entertain them
in the first place, dear
life, friend.
Don't leave me here without you.

Thanks Prayer at the Cove

A year ago today
I was unable to speak
one syntactically coherent
thought let alone write it down: today
in this dear and absurdly allegorical place
by your grace
I am here
and now in that graveyard, its skyline
visible not from the November leaflessness
and I am here to say
it's 5 o'clock, too late to write more
(especially for the one whose eyes
are starting to get dark), the single
dispirited swan out on the windless brown
transparent floor floating
gradually backward
blackward
no this is what I still
can see, white
as a joint in a box of little cigars—
and where is mate
Lord, it is almost winter in the year
2000 and now I look up to find five
practically unseeable mallards at my feet
they have crossed
nearly standing on earth they're so close
looking up to me
for bread—
that's what my eyes of flesh see (barely)
but what I wished to say
is this, listen:
a year ago today
I found myself riding the subway psychotic
(I wasn't depressed, I wanted to rip my face off)
unable to write what I thought, which was nothing
though I tried though I finally stopped trying and looked up
at the face of the man directly across from me, and it began
to melt before my eyes
and in an instant it was young again
the face he must have had

once when he was five
and in an instant it happened again only this time
it changed to the face of his elderly
corpse and back in time
it changed
to his face at our present
moment of time's flowing and then
as if transparently
superimposed I saw them all at once
OK I was insane but how insane
can someone be I thought, I did not
know you then
I didn't know you were there God
(that's what we call you, grunt grunt)
as you are at every moment
everywhere of what we call
the future and the past
And then I tried once more
experimentally
I focused on another's face, no need to describe it
there is only one
underneath
these scary and extremely
realistic rubber masks
and there is as I also know now
by your grace one
and only one person on earth
beneath a certain depth
the terror and the love
are one, like hunger, same
in everyone
and it happened again, das Unglück geschah
you might say nur mir allein it happened
no matter who I looked at
for maybe five minutes long enough
long enough
this hidden trinity
I saw, the others
will say I am making it up
as if that mattered
Lord,
I make up nothing
not one word.

David Baker

(1954–)

Hyper

Then a stillness descended the blue hills.
I say stillness. They were three deer, then four.
They crept down the old bean field, these four deer,
for fifteen minutes—more—as we watched them

in the field, in the soughing snow. That's how
slowly they moved in stillness, slender deer.
The fourth limped behind the other three,
we could see, even in the darkness, as it

dragged its right hindquarter where it was
hit or shot. Katie sat back on her heels.
The dog held in his prints, or Kate held him,
hardly breathing at first. Then we relaxed.

Blue night descended our neighbor's blown hills.
And the calm that comes with seeing something
beautiful but far from perfect descended—
absolute attention, a fixity.

I say absolute. It was stillness.

In the books we gathered, the first theory
holds that the condition's emergence is
most common at age eight, if less in girls
than boys, or more vividly seen in boys
whose fidgets, whose deficit attentions,
like little psycho-economic realms,
are prone to twitches-turned-to-virulence,
anxieties palpable in vocalized
explosions—though now we know in girls
it's only on the surface less severe,

which explains her months of bubbling tension,
her long blue drifts and snowy distractions.
I say distractions. Of course I mean how,
clinically, tyrosine hydroxylase
activity—the "rate limiting enzyme
dopamine synthesis"—disrupts, burns,
then rewires her brain's chemical pathways.

Let me put it another way. After
twenty-four math problems, the twenty-fifth
still baffles her, pencil gnawed, eraser-
scuff-shadows like black veins on her homework.

It's not just the theory of division
she no longer gets, it's her hot clothes, her
itchy ear, the ruby-throated hummingbird's
picture on the fridge, what's in the fridge, whose

socks these are, why, until I'm exhausted
and yell again. Until she's gone away
to her room, lights off, to sulk, read, cry, draw.
No longer trusting to memory, she

writes everything in her journal now, then
ties it with a broken strand of necklace.
Of her friends: *I am the funny one.* Mom:
She has red hair and freckles to. Under Dad:

I have his bad temper. I know. I looked.

In one sketch she finished, just before we
learned what was wrong—I mean, before we knew
what to call what was wrong, how to treat it,
how to treat *her*—she captured her favorite
cat with a skill that skips across my chest.
He's on a throw rug, asleep. The rug's fringe
ruffles just so. The measure of her love is
visible in each delicate stroke, from
his fetal repose, ears down, eyes sealed
softly, paws curled inward, to the tiger lines
of his coat deepened by thick textures
where she's slightly rubbed away the contours

with her thumb to winter coat gray. He's soft,
he's purring, he's utterly relaxed asleep.
One day, before we learned what was wrong,
she taped it to a pillow on my bed.
Terry Is Tired she'd printed at the top.

How many ways do we measure things by
what they're not. I say things. Mostly her mind
is going too fast, yet the doctors give her,
I'm not kidding, amphetamines—

speed, we used to say, when we needed it—
Ritalin, which wears off hard and often,
Adderal, which lasts all day though her food's
untouched and sleep comes late. The irony

is the medicine slows her down. She pays
attention, understands things. The theory
is, AD/HD patients "aren't hyper-
aroused, they're underaroused," so they lurch

and hurtle forward, hungry for focus.
Another theory says the brain's two lobes
are missized. Their circuits "lose their balance."
One makes much of handedness—left—red hair,

allergies, wan skin, an Irish past . . .

We watched four deer in stillness walking there.
Stillness walking, like the young blue deer hurt
but beautiful. In her theory of
division, Katie's started drawing them—
her rendering's reduced them down to three.
She has carefully lined the cut bean rows
in contours like the dog's brushed coat. Snowflakes
dot the winter paper. Two small deer stand
alert on either side of the hurt one
leaning now to bite the season's dried-up stems.
Their ears are perched like hands, noses up, tails
tufted in a hundred tiny pencil lines.
She's been hunkered over her drawing pad,
humming, for an hour. So I watch. I say

watch. I ask why she's made the little hurt
one so big. Silly. He's not hurt that bad,
she says. She doesn't look up. That one's you.

∽

Melancholy Man

1.

What makes Robert Burton's Anatomy of Melancholy
so hard to put down is his wild branching rhetoric.
It's not enough to race pathologies of mind, whatever
path a lost mind takes—he wants to make it rhyme,
invest it with the kind of power music makes or minds
in a quandary, and give it memory's crutch mnemonics.
Ingress, progress, regress, egress, much alike, he writes,

citing four culpable causes of "discontents, cares,
miseries, etc.," yet even here his rhyming trochees
don't suffice as art until he finishes the sentence
with a flourish suitable to the Bible or beloved Lucretius:
*blindness seizeth on us in the beginning, labour
in the middle, grief in the end, error in all.*
Root to trunk to limb to leaf—as he might say.

2.

In my friend's voice I hear a ghost.
Home from the hospital, he is, at sixty-two,
scared of his heart's heredity—who wouldn't be?—
a host of uncles dead before their time, his father,
at fifty-six, the four chambers of whose heart
filled with the effluvium of both their lifetimes.
He feels the line stretching to him the way

the branching tree leads or leans, one to the next,
the way the heart goes bad one tapped vein at a time.
Melancholy man, he calls himself, though he has written
of a cloud, even of peaceable clouds in a painting,

it is right to think of these as elegies of the spirit, to see
their forms as melancholy hosts, and the poet watching
clouds is watching phantoms levitating stone.

   3.

How hard to hold to a single thought in hand.
Sorrow is one cause but confusion itself is symptom
of the malady—Burton's explanations being one part
medicine, one part art, and clearly confessional
of his brooding mind. I say *fickle, fugitive, they may
not abide to tarry in one place long. Eftsoons pleased,
and anon displeased, as a man that's bitten with fleas.*

Love of learning, he says, is a central cause,
as is, among "accidental sources," too much education.
Thus the sore afflicted go commonly meditating
unto themselves, thus they sit, abrood, aloof, aloft,
senseless to nature and time, and in hopes to recover
must turn rustic, rude, or melancholize alone.
But how hard not to be enchanted with the rhyme.

   4.

When his best friend died, at fifty-five, the good heart
deserted its host. It's in his voice, spectral, static
on the line. The heartline of the graph draws
straight to him. Loss of friends is so great a cause,
Burton says, *amongst the Pagan Indians, their wives
and servants voluntarily die with them.*
He sees Bill's ghost, cold, candle-white,

and like a cloud grown abstract—though none of us dies
entirely, he writes, through some of us, all of us sometimes
come back sapling, seedling, cell, like second growth,
he finds himself alone, dead weight of his bones,
standing over graves in moonlight's shadow.
He hears his pulse beat in his ear. Pressed hard,
he says, against the receiver, to see—are you still here?

Michael Lauchlan

(1954–)

What You Hadn't

One pain forgives another;
mashed thumb obliterates headache.
Malaria returned, dragged your liver
with all your other failures
           from that ugly flat
where you burned so many pots of stew
and chased your daughter's beaus away.
"If we hadn't lost the house," I might say now,
or "if you hadn't driven the car
onto the basketball court."
           But there you sat,
dozed, watched the televised war,
the burn scar from the barrel of the B.A.R.
warning me not to be a softy.
Then you wept to the skinny boy
you pressed against it into your vast belly,
against your sweat and breath,
saying, "Never touch a gun."
           So desperate,
cursed to drink by birth and war,
beaten, slicing ham and cutting steaks
in a disappointing sixties,
you'd nothing left to give a boy
but a clip with the shells dumped out.

Joe Bolton

(1961–1990)

Laguna Beach Breakdown

You had come searching for a second chance,
But trying to break through, merely broke down,
Until at last any sense of purpose
Seemed nothing more than something else to lose.
You let it go and, seeing no reason to mourn
What you could no longer name, kept silence
Under the vast vacuum of a heaven.
Someone had nailed stars up to hold in place.
You were hoping maybe a change of season
Might help, but there was none. You woke at dawn
Shuddering in the indifferent embrace
Of your own arms, unable to turn or return,
Dreaming of drowning, neutral as seaweed in the war
The sea continually waged against the shore.

A Couple of Suicide Cases

1

"What could have possessed him?" people later
    will say. "He had his whole life
ahead of him."—that *him* being Jimmy Barlow,
    eighteen, attendant
at the Texaco on Highway 68 in Draffenville,
    who, come to dusk, is going to
drive the ten miles to Kentucky Dam, park
    his beaten Datsun, stroll

out onto the high concrete platform, gaze awhile
    at the first stars, at the last light
leaving the river, then casually—as if it were
    the most natural thing
in the world—jump, like a baby into the basket
    of its mother's open arms.
And in that split second before gravity
    gets hold of him, before
the water like a supercooled unbreathable air
    rushes up to take him,
he, Jimmy Barlow, will feel entirely free
    for the first time in his life.

    2
"Goddamnsonofabitchingcocksuckingmotherfuckingasslicking-
    bastards"
    That's what Pat said when he broke down
the door to the roof of Kincannon Hall at Ole Miss, breaking
    his hand in the process. He didn't care:
he was a drunk ex-boxer from New York City, and flunking out.
    We were all drunk, too, following him like
disciples over the pebbles-frozen-in-tar surface—to watch
    the sunrise, to keep him from jumping.
We sat down beside him on the ledge facing east, unsteady,
    dangling our legs over the seven-story drop.
After a while, the stars began to pale in a sky that seemed
    suddenly huge, and then the horizon
was flowing through and through itself, like a watercolor
    in progress. Houses, fields, woods
came forward in fog. The world's dew turned into our sweat.
    It was May 1980 in Oxford, Mississippi.
We were young, drunk, ready to take on the whole South.
    There was no telling what might happen.
"Goddamnsonofabitchingcocksuckingmotherfuckingasslicking-
    bastards,"
    Pat said to the campus policemen who soon arrived.

Kelly Ann Malone

(1963–)

Devices on Standby

I've tucked away two forty-fours.
They're deep within a wall.
Their bullets line my dresser drawers
and wait for me to call.

Two vials filled with cyanide
are safe within their space.
I've stashed them in a pot outside
beneath the Queen Anne's lace.

Two gleaming knives to slit my wrists
sit nestled in a shed.
I'll use them if my grief persists
to soak my ivory bed.

Two slipknots made of sturdy rope
sit limp upon a chair.
It helps me when I cannot cope
to know that they are there.

You ask me why they come in two's?
the need for added stress?
In case the first one that I choose
is launched without success.

I've had these items in my house
for over forty years.
I've hid them from my kids and spouse,
my neighbors and my peers.

I tried to do it years ago,
but then I had a boy.

And two more children in a row,
brought intermittent joy.

At last I thought my work was done,
and I could end my life.
But now my daughter has a son,
my son now has a wife.

I'll get around to my demise
and give in to despair,
when I can look into their eyes
and tell them I don't care.

Brian Turner

(1967–)

Eulogy

It happens on a Monday, at 11:20 A.M.,
as tower guards eat sandwiches
and seagulls drift by on the Tigris River.
Prisoners tilt their heads to the west
though burlap sacks and duct tape blind them.
The sound reverberates down concertina coils
the way piano wire thrums when given slack.
And it happens like this, on a blue day of sun,
when Private Miller pulls the trigger
to take brass and fire into his mouth:
the sound lifts the birds up off the water,
a mongoose pauses under the orange trees,
and nothing can stop it now, no matter what
blur of motion surrounds him, no matter what voices
crackle over the radio in static confusion,
because if only for this moment the earth is stilled,
and Private Miller has found what low hush there is
down in the eucalyptus shade, there by the river.

PFC B. Miller
(1980–March 22, 2003)

Kevin Young

(1970–)

Coke® (The Real Thing)

His nose
is open—
he wants him

some white
girl, needs
to score—

Might want
to quit
her, but he's

an addick
& she's his dealer
& only takes

ten percent.
Says she'll hook
him up with Warhol—*White*

lines Blowin through
my mind
And now I'm having

fun baby—
Don't be so nosy,
he's got it under

control. Just a chippie.
Needs advice like another
hole in his nose—

done a job
on it already.
Snowed. Nose

blown & eroded
like the Sphinx,
his olfactory's gone

on strike
—to pot—scabs
brought in. White

collared crime.
Bidnessman is caught
with 17 kilos He's out
on bail & out of jail
& that's the way it goes—
On fire, cranks

out work
—Prometheus, epidermis—
ALAS; "WINGS"

MOSTLY BUZZARDS—
culture vultures
who swoop & swallow

studios whole,
day after day. *Huh—*
sugar—cane—

Some leave out
his place
with paint not dry

others give bills
he burns by
the hundreds

taking a lighter
to Ben Franklin's
face, kite flying

lightening. He's over
it all, pours
a still

life, basket
of nuts & fruit,
birdfood

dumped on the head
of the collector showing
off her black

chaffeur. Rochester—
Freeze—Rock—
smoke & mirrors

the funhouse
he snorts off—the dollar
the razor—dusted.

from *In the Realms of the Unreal: "Insane" Writings*

(John G. H. Oakes, editor)
(published 1991)

Nicol

By My Own Hand

I watched these
cold stiff fingers
reach in searching
the sacred edge
the sharp undoing
and I didn't struggle
against them
as a long thin line
appeared
above the throbbing
and the sweet red wine
spilled over
and mixed itself together
with the bitter
of salty tears
and once again I lay
in this frothy soup
never knowing
what's to come of it
because I was
unable to bear
the best of it

from *In the Realms of the Unreal:*
"Insane" Writings

(John G. H. Oakes, editor)
(published 1991)

Richard Beard

The Queen's Foreboding

Intimations of Dementia / Gertrud's prebirth

to let be or to not let be:
the prickly thorn of questing
all's too numb, dumbly askings
who's well who ends ill, before
issue of protests, portents and pretends;
'tis not of this world, this whelp
within my womb, knows where to prod
exactly on the tender foreknowledge
of vainglory's wonderings whamming
witchy whoo's owllike smuttings
besmirched within a belly's full
wailing already for the dark corridor
of entrance in and exit out, the re-
capitulation, nights' capricious giving-
in to the throne's dementia and demands
for princely conduct toward an ill-
defined need of hairy whooze and heir-
looms the size of pinpoints beginning
kingdoms-cometo loose this madness
on us all: God or gods befouled
by discordant desires and divine right,
whole destinies determined in the toss
of sickly seed, doubled by doldrums
(fishy and dunmarked) deeded rightly
and practiced nightly until this, now
a weighty waiting-in, thrashing within
an eternal doubt, deeped in a seeping
sac of unborn bones and hair and doom:

which way one turns, the lump is ever there,
and blood shall curdle on this moment's notice
of what has passed and shall yet pass
and crones know more than mother, while
mother wiles hours, as the obligatory ½
pleasure swells fullblown in the destiny
of bloody dust's insistence on his kingdom.

this alien madness crouching ready in me
kin of sodden saints worth but sick damns,
my profit no mere lamb, a sham seen slick,
with prophet's spoonfed ways, an offscene
stab in darkness, demon dancing on the edge
of bubbling tubs, stirring all the mucks
of aging sadness, growing forcefully to know
the mad why's of this his first decision:
letit go, let it be, Godbless,
and let him know the scrambly fixings
of one mother's obeying the obstructions
of queenly duty, you shall pay as you've
paid me, and kick and roll and moan
and madden, as my poor poor surrogate floats
down Lethe with pale flowers in her dead mouth.

Jeff Holt

(1971–)

Imbalance

Echoing threats drown out the quiet roar
Of lattes, strangers laughing easily.
My thoughts are flopping fishes, cold, not sure
That water will return. I barely see
Past trembling fingers I still recognize
By bitten nails, that scab. Wait. Did I speak?
My limbs are clown balloons. I need to rise,
Smile as I leave. Today I will not break.

I will not brake once I am out that door;
I'll race across charred ruins, fly through Hell—
Slow down. I am a paying customer
At Border's; so what if I'm not feeling well?
Strangers can't hear the threats, that doctor said.
I rise, cling to his words, stalk through these dead.

The Patient

The doctors know I dream when I'm awake.
I've smoked until my fingertips are brown.
Watching the door, I sit alone and shake.

My sister and her kids, Kelly and Jake,
Played games with me when I'd sink this far down
Until they knew I dream when I'm awake.

When Beth comes now, her smile is bright and fake.
She doesn't want to bring the kids downtown.
She leaves too soon. I sit alone and shake.

The voice is back. It whispers till I ache.
I'm soaked in sweat and tangled in my gown
When they catch me dreaming while still awake.

They've brought more pills that they must watch me take.
They're lifeguards staring at me as I drown.
They leave again. I sit alone and shake.

I'm stuck in a glass bubble I can't break.
The others stand outside and watch the clown.
I wish I didn't dream when I'm awake.
The room grows dark. I sit alone and shake.

Ricky Cantor

(1985–)

E 9th Street

I'm from mental illnesses and corner bars
and taking parts from stolen cars.

I'm from street fights at three thirty
and ass whipping 'til next morning.

I'm from a drunken father and a pissed off mother
and was raised by my older sister and brother.

I'm from parents that are Mexican
and I'm ashamed to say that I'm American.

I'm from hard boiled eggs and government cheese
oh, and did I mention ass beating.

I'm from joyrides at five
and a brother that loves to say access denied.

I'm from a little sister who's worst than crazy
and two little brothers that are fucking lazy.

Coda

Anne Stevenson

(1933–)

Letter to Sylvia Plath

They are great healers, English springs.
You loved their delicate colourings—
sequential yellows, eggshell blues—
not pigments you preferred to use,
lady of pallors and foetal jars
and surgical interiors.
But wasn't it warmth you wanted most?

These Grantchester willows keep your ghost,
young and in love and half way through
the half-life that was left to you.
The Cam still crawls through patient grass,
preserving ephemerals in glass.
A bull thrush shouts from a willow thicket,
Catch it! Catch it! Catch it! Catch it!
Catch what? An owl in a petalled dress?
The gnarl at the root of a distress?

Dear Sylvia, we must close our book.
Three springs you've perched like a black rook
between sweet weather and my mind.
At last I have to seem unkind
and exorcise my awkward awe.
My shoulder doesn't like your claw.

Yet first, forgiveness. Let me shake
some echoes from old balled eyed Blake
over your grave and praise in rhyme
the fiercest poet of our time—

you with your outsized gift for joy
who did the winged life destroy,
and bought with death a mammoth name
to set in the cold museum of fame.

Your art was darkness. No, your art
was a gulping candle in the dark.
In the beginning was a curse:
a hag, a drowned man and a nurse
hid in the mirror of the moon
unquietly to work your doom.
A dissolute nun, you had to serve
the demon muse who peeled your nerve
and fuelled your energy with hate.
Malevolent will-power made you great,
while round you in the Sacred Wood
tall archetypal statues stood
rooted in air and in your mind.
The proud impossibles loomed behind,
pilasters buttressing a frieze
of marble, moonlit amputees.

Sylvia, I see you in this view
of glassy absolutes where you,
a frantic Alice, trip on snares,
crumple and drown in your own tears.
You were your cave of crippled dreams
and ineradicable screams,
and you were the pure gold honey bee
prisoned in poisonous jealousy.

The gratitude and love you thought
the world would give you if you fought
for all your tears could not be found
in reputation's building ground.
O give the mole an eagle's soul
and watch it battling in its hole.

Because you were selfish and sad and died,
we have grown up on the other side
of a famous girl you didn't know.
The future is where the dead go

in rage, bewilderment and pain
to make and magnify their name.

Meanwhile, the continuous present casts
longer reflections on the past.
Nothing has changed much. Famine, war
fatten your Spider as before.
Your hospital of bleeding parts
devours its haul of human hearts,
excreting what it cannot use
as celluloid or paper news;
eye for eye and tooth for tooth,
bomb for bomb and youth for youth.

Yet who would believe the colour green
had so many ways of being green?
In England, still, your poet's spring
arrives, unravelling everything.
A yellowhammer in the gorse
creates each minute's universe;
a blackbird singing from a thorn
is all the joy of being reborn.

Even in Heptonstall in May
the wind invites itself away,
leaving black stone to compromise
with stitchwort, dandelions and flies.
Tell me, do all those weeds and trees
strewing their cool longevities
over the garden of your bed
have time for you, now you are dead?

Behind the pricked-out drape of night
is there a sheet-white screen of light
where death meets birth to reconcile
the contradictions of your will?
Perfection is terrible, you said.
The perfect are barren, like the dead.

Yet life, more terrible, maunches on,
as blood-red light loops back at dawn,
seizing, devouring, giving birth

to the mass atrocity of the earth.
Poor Sylvia, could you not have been
a little smaller than a queen—
a river, not a tidal wave
engulfing all you tried to save?

Rather than not be justified
you sickened in loneliness and died,
while we live on in messy lives,
rueful or tired or barely wise.
Ageing, we labour to exist.
Beyond existence, nothing is.
Out of this world there is no source
of yellower rape or golder gorse,
nor in the galaxy higher place,
I think, for human mind or face.

We learn to be human when we kneel
to imagination, which is real
long after reality is dead
and history has put its bones to bed.
Sylvia, you have won at last,
embodying the living past,
catching the anguish of your age
in accents of a private rage.

Biographical Notes on the Poets

Matthew Arnold (1822–1888)
Arnold was born in Laleham-on-Thames, the son of Dr. Thomas Arnold, a renowned and influential teacher, headmaster of the Rugby School, and later a professor at Oxford. Arnold attended Rugby, where he also later taught, and subsequently Balliol College, Oxford. In 1847 he became secretary to Lord Lansdowne, and shortly after, he began publishing both criticism and poetry, initially under the pseudonym "A." He was named professor of poetry at Oxford in 1858.

Jimmy Santiago Baca (1952–)
Baca was born in New Mexico of Native American and Hispanic descent. His father died from complications of alcohol use, and his mother left him in the care of his grandparents, who subsequently sent him tot an orphanage. He dropped out of school and ran away at the age of thirteen, adapting to life on the street. At age twenty-one he was incarcerated for drug-related charges and was given a six-year prison term in Arizona. It was during his time in prison that Baca taught himself how to read and started to write poetry. On encouragement from an inmate, he sent his work to *Mother Jones* magazine in San Francisco. He came to the attention of the editor, who helped him publish his first book while Baca was still in prison. In 1979 he was released from prison. He continues to write and to lead workshops and teach across the country in public high schools, universities, housing projects, and prisons.

David Baker (1954–)
Baker was born in Maine and grew up in Missouri. He attended Central Missouri State University for his bachelor's and master's degrees.

Baker served as editor for the University of Utah's *Quarterly West* while earning a Ph.D. at that school. He subsequently taught at the University of Utah, Kenyon College, and Cornell University, and he currently teaches at Denison University in Ohio.

John Codrington Bampfylde (1754–1796)
Bampfylde was born in Devon and grew up on a farm. He attended Cambridge University and subsequently moved to London where he fell in love with the Marchioness Thomond and wrote her sixteen sonnets. These, with three other poems, are the entirety of his published work. When his proposal for marriage was rejected by the girl's uncle, he broke the windows of the uncle's house in rage and was incarcerated in Newgate Prison. His family bailed him out, but he was soon moved to a private asylum in Chelsea where he spent most of the next seven years. He died of consumption in 1796.

Mary Barber (c. 1690–c. 1757)
Barber was born in England and married an Irishman. She had four children and began to publish in Dublin, with the Carteret family as benefactors. In 1728, Jonathan Swift began to finance her poetry. Swift sent Barber to England to promote her work. Though her work was well received, she returned to Ireland in 1732. In 1747 she became ill and ceased publishing.

Alexander Barclay (1475–1552)
Barclay grew up in Croydon and attended Oriel College, Oxford. Thereafter he served as chaplain at Ottery St. Mary College, Devonshire. In 1513 he entered the monastery of Ely as a monk.

Elizabeth Barrett Browning (1806–1861)
Barrett Browning was born in Durham into a large, wealthy family. She was well schooled, but at age fourteen she suffered lung problems, and the following year, a serious back injury, followed by signs of nervous instability by age twenty. She was treated with both morphine and opium, drugs that she continued using for the remainder of her life. Her resources and education were extensive, and she had an extremely close relationship with her father. She published first anonymously

and then by 1838 under her own name. The Barretts moved to London, but after her two brothers died in accidents Elizabeth became house-bound for five years. During this time she produced *Poems*, which caught the eye of Robert Browning upon its publication. Robert and Elizabeth wrote numerous love sonnets and letters and finally eloped in 1846 to Florence, where Elizabeth became healthy enough to have a son and continued writing. She was never reconciled with her father and died in Florence at age fifty-five.

R. L. Barth (1947–)

Barth describes being "educated in the Marine Corps (with advanced studies in Vietnam)" and at Northern Kentucky State University and Stanford University. He is the author of *Looking for Peace, A Soldier's Time*, and *Deeply Dug In* as well as the editor of *The Selected Poems of Yvor Winters, The Selected Poems of Janet Lewis*, and *The Selected Letters of Yvor Winters*. He lives with his wife, Susan, in Kentucky, where he continues to work on a sequence of poems about the Battle of Dien Bien Phu.

Thomas Haynes Bayly (1797–1839)

Bayly was born in Bath, England, to parents from well-respected fami-lies. He attended the Winchester School, where he ran their weekly newspaper. On a trip to Dublin, Bayly began to experiment with writing ballads and poetry, which were published in England starting in 1824. In 1826 he married a wealthy Irish woman, with whom he had three children. His son died at the age of six, and his wife's property was handled poorly, leaving them in debt. Bayly wrote numerous plays and two novels but was unable to gain financial stability, and he began to lose his health at a young age. He died at the age of forty-two.

Thomas P. Beresford (1946–)

Beresford is professor of psychiatry at the University of Colorado. He received his undergraduate degree from Stanford University and his medical degree from the University of Colorado. After psychiatric residency at Harvard, he received his master's degree from Boston College and won a Stegner Fellowship in poetry, studying with Kenneth Fields and the late Henri Coulette. He has published two chapbooks (Robert L. Barth Press) and has had poems published in a variety of literary and medical journals. His literary essays have appeared in

The Southern Review and *The Pharos*. As a clinical scientist he has authored four books and more than 120 research articles.

John Berryman (1914–1972)

Berryman was born in Oklahoma to a banker and a school teacher. They moved to Florida, and when Berryman was eleven years old his father committed suicide. His mother remarried, and the family moved to New York City. Berryman studied at Columbia University and spent two years at Cambridge University, where he met Yeats and Dylan Thomas (q.v.). He taught at Harvard and at the University of Minnesota. He consistently battled depression and alcoholism, for which he was hospitalized on several occasions. At age fifty-seven Berryman ended his life by jumping off a bridge in Minneapolis.

Elizabeth Bishop (1911–1979)

Bishop was born in Worcester, Massachusetts. When she was eight months old her father died and her mother entered an asylum, where she remained for the rest of her life. Bishop was raised by her grandparents in Nova Scotia and Massachusetts, and she missed much of grade school because of lung ailments. She graduated from Vassar, and on a trip to Brazil she fell in love with a Brazilian woman, Lota de Macedo Soares. They lived and traveled together until ill health and an overdose of pills led to de Macedo's death. Bishop was a contemporary of the confessional poets and a close confidante and friend of Robert Lowell (q.v.). Unlike Lowell and their confessional contemporaries, Bishop's work displays little emotional self-disclosure, but evidence from a variety of sources indicates that Bishop struggled with alcohol and depression. The poem included in this anthology likely derives from her trips to St. Elizabeths, a federal psychiatric hospital in Washington, DC, where she visited Ezra Pound, who was held there by reason of insanity for treasonous actions during World War II.

William Blake (1757–1827)

Blake was born into poverty in London and learned to read and write at home. He attended the Royal Academy of Arts and, after an apprenticeship with a local artist, attempted to establish his own engraving business. At twenty-three, Blake married Catherine Boucher, who was uneducated and poor. After teaching her to read and write, they began painting and binding his first books together. From a young age he experienced visions and communications with spirits, and during his adult life he endured long periods of depression. Blake was not widely recognized as an artist or a poet during his lifetime. His first collection of poetry was not published until 1905.

Robert Bloomfield (1766–1823)
Bloomfield, the son of a tailor and a schoolteacher, was born in Honington, Suffolk. His father died when Bloomfield was one year old. At five feet tall and too frail for farm work, he was sent to London to learn shoemaking from his brother. He is reputed to have composed poems in his head while cobbling, writing them down later and eventually publishing the fourteen-hundred-line "The Farmer's Boy" to some critical and popular acclaim. In this Romantic era, his literary acclaim in part derived from his "poet-cobbler" persona, sharing features of the early life of John Clare (q.v.) in his involvement in but disjunction from literary society. Throughout his life, Bloomfield's financial security waxed and waned, and though he continued to publish into his later years, he died destitute.

Robert Bly (1926–)
Bly was born into a farming family in Madison, Minnesota. He served in the U.S. Navy for two years before entering St. Olaf College. After a year he transferred to Harvard, where he graduated with highest honors in 1950. His studies had shifted from medicine to English, and among his classmates were John Ashbury, Adrienne Rich, and Frank O'Hara. He lived for six months in a cabin in Minnesota after college and then moved to New York City, writing and working part-time to make ends meet. For two years he attended the University of Iowa Writers' Workshop and married writer Carol McLean just before his graduation in 1956. The two returned to his farm in Minnesota before Bly traveled on a Fulbright fellowship to Norway, his family's country of origin, where he began to translate Scandinavian poetry. Upon his return to Minnesota, he began a literary magazine called *The Fifties*, later changed to take the name *The Sixties*. His political activities have included activism against the Vietnam War and work toward the establishment of a "Men's Movement" to complement the Women's Movement. He was divorced and remarried, and currently resides on his farm in Minnesota.

Louise Bogan (1897–1970)

Bogan was born in Livermore Falls, Maine. At the age of eight she was sent to the Boston Girls' Latin School and then attended Boston University for one year in 1915, having already planned a career in writing. She published her first volume of poetry at age twenty-two and made her living as a freelance literary critic. She married the writer Raymond Holden in 1925, but this relationship ended in divorce. Her circle of literary colleagues included William Carlos Williams, Edmund Wilson, and Theodore Roethke (q.v.). In 1931 she secured a long-term job at the *New Yorker* as a poetry critic. She continually battled depression, for which she was hospitalized twice.

Joseph Bolton (1961–1990)

Bolton was born in Cadiz, Kentucky, and spent his childhood in that state, where his parents were teachers. After a year on scholarship at the University of Mississippi, Bolton returned to Kentucky and received his undergraduate degree at Western Kentucky University. He pursued an MFA in writing at the University of Arizona, and then attended writing programs in Houston, at the University of Florida, Gainesville, and at the University of Arizona. Upon completion of his program at Arizona, he compiled a poetry collection from his thesis. The next day he committed suicide, leaving no explanation.

Anne Bradstreet (1612–1672)

Bradstreet was born in England to a wealthy family. Her father moved the family to America when she was only eighteen to become governor of the Puritan settlement of Massachusetts. She had been married at sixteen to Simon Bradstreet, who accompanied them and subsequently served as governor. In America, Bradstreet wrote poetry for her immediate friends and family while rearing eight children and maintaining a busy and high-profile colonial household. Her brother-in-law brought her poems to England, where they were published with some success in 1650, though most were published posthumously in America.

Robert Bridges (1844–1930)

Bridges was born in Upper Walmer, Kent, into a large family. His father died when he was nine years old, and the following year he began his studies at Eton. In 1863 he matriculated at Corpus Christi College, Oxford, intrigued by poetry but planning to enter the clergy.

At Oxford he became lifelong friends with Gerard Manley Hopkins (q.v.). Also while at university Bridges was deeply affected by the death of his brother. He graduated in 1867, and shortly thereafter while traveling to Jerusalem he learned that his sister and her family had been murdered in England. In 1869 Bridges entered medical school at St. Bartholomew's Hospital and subsequently worked at La Pitié Hospital in Paris. He stopped working as a physician after a severe bout of pneumonia in 1881, and devoted himself to writing. In 1884 he married Monica Waterhouse, with whom he had three children. In 1913 he was named poet laureate, and he later received honorary doctorates from Columbia University, the University of Michigan, and Harvard University.

Robert Burton (1577–1640)

Burton was born in Lindley, Leicestershire, and attended Brasenose College, Oxford. During this time there is an unexplained break in his studies; interestingly, the only record of his name during this period is in the journals of Simon Forman, a physician who recorded a patient by the name of Robert Burton diagnosed with "melancholy." In 1599 he reenrolled at Oxford, this time at Christ Church, where he attained his degree. He remained to work as a priest paid through the Oxford church of St. Thomas. He wrote verse and a number of plays in his lifetime, but his best-known contribution to literature and medicine is his mammoth prose work, *The Anatomy of Melancholy*. This tome, with its verse "Abstract" as an introduction, was initially published in 1621 and underwent a number of revisions, with each succeeding edition larger than the last.

George Gordon, Lord Byron (1788–1824)

Byron was born into nobility. Despite a congenitally deformed foot, he pursued academics and sports ambitiously as a youth. He attended Harrow School at Harrow-on-the-Hill and Trinity College, Cambridge. He squandered large amounts of money, and after numerous love affairs and a failed marriage, he left England in 1815 never to return. He first settled briefly in Geneva, where he became friends with the poet Percy Bysshe Shelley (q.v.), and then lived for a time in Venice, Italy. When the Greek War of Independence against Turkey broke out, Byron devoted himself to the Greek cause, both providing financial support and joining the forces himself. He died in Greece, at the age of thirty-six, though not in combat. The exact cause of his death is unknown, though it was likely related to infection and a fever complicated by leech treatment. Torquato Tasso, the subject of Byron's "Lament," was a sixteenth-century poet subject to periods of behavioral instability and was at one point committed to an asylum.

Ricky Cantor (1985–)

Cantor was born and raised in Brooklyn, New York, and lives in Providence, Rhode Island. For three years, Cantor has participated in New Urban Arts, a nationally recognized interdisciplinary art studio for high school students (www.newurbanarts.org), where he has worked with artist mentors in writing poetry. He first started writing in elementary school when a counselor gave him a notebook and told him to write down everything that went on each day. His poems have appeared in *FLIP* (May 2005 and May 2006), an annual zine publication by New Urban Arts, and *Muzine*, "the uncensored voice of Rhode Island youth," a publication by AS220 (vols. 22 and 23). "E 9th Street" was first published in *Thinking Hurts*, an anthology of poetry by high school students at New Urban Arts (December 2005).

James Carkesse (birth/death dates unknown; published 1679)

Carkesse was educated at Westminster and entered Christ Church, Oxford, on a scholarship in 1652. He was subsequently elected to the Royal Society and worked as a clerk in the Navy Office under Samuel Pepys. He married, but lacked financial stability, and was eventually found guilty of bribery and theft. Though he was discharged from his position, he apparently threatened his way back into work but was subsequently committed to Bedlam asylum in 1678 for, among other symptoms, religious delusions. While in Bedlam, Carkesse became the first English poet to publish while institutionalized. He was moved to a small private asylum in Finsbury under the care of Dr. Thomas Allen. However, Carkesse periodically became quite violent and had to be returned to Bedlam, at times under high security, where he was administered "physicks" and sometimes held in darkness. Much of what is known of Carkesse comes from the reports of his many, and often prominent, visitors who knew of him initially through his poetry.

Hayden Carruth (1921–)

Carruth was born in Connecticut and attended the University of North Carolina. He served in World War II in the U.S. Army Air Corps in Italy.

He went on to study and work as an editor at the University of Chicago and then in New York. In 1953 he was admitted to the Westchester Division of New York Hospital, formerly Bloomingdale Asylum, where he spent fifteen months as an inpatient. He has subsequently written explicitly about his battles with depression, anxiety, suicidality, and alcohol.

Margaret Cavendish, Duchess of Newcastle (c. 1624–1674)

Cavendish was born into a wealthy Royalist family. Her father died when she was two, and when she was sixteen the political turmoil leading to the Civil War forced her family to leave England with Charles I. Cavendish became a maid of honor in the court of Queen Henrietta Maria and was subsequently exiled a second time with this court to France in 1644. She left the court when she met William Cavendish, whom she married in 1645. She returned to England in 1651 with a brother-in-law to attempt to establish her husband's rights to an estate as the Duke of Newcastle. At this time she began to publish, financed by her husband, though he remained in exile until 1665. Unusual for a woman, she participated in the Royal Society of London, corresponded extensively with philosophers such as Hobbes and Descartes, and maintained an active interest in science and scientific theory.

Thomas Chatterton (1752–1770)

Chatterton grew up in Bristol and was home-schooled, learning to read from the Bible. He apprenticed as a scribe in Bristol and began a promising career as a poet, moving to London at age seventeen. Soon, however, he lost all motivation, appetite, and, eventually, desire to live. He was found dead in his bed four months after his arrival. Medical inquest identified arsenic as the agent and suicide as the cause. However, modern scholarship has suggested that the arsenic poisoning may have been accidental, possibly related to treatment for a sexually transmitted disease.

John Clare (1793–1864)

Clare was born in Northamptonshire into an indigent family. He worked on a farm in his childhood and was given leave for three months a year to learn to read and write in town. He began to write poetry as a child, and in 1820 his poetry was discovered by a Stamford bookseller. Shortly after, he received a salary from literary benefactors; he published his first book and married that same year. This book, primarily about rural life, was to be the most successful during his lifetime, and earned him a reputation as a "peasant-poet." He reacted with annoyance at being considered an oddity, but appreciated the positive reception of his poetry; however, he failed at his plan to support his family by writing, and began to drink heavily. He experienced frequent bouts of depression and had been tormented since childhood by fainting spells and nightmares associated with having seen a man fall from a load of hay and break his neck. In 1837 he was placed in High Beech, a private asylum. He remained institutionalized there, suffering misconceptions about his identity, until 1841 when he walked eight miles home to Northampshire. He was sent afterward to Northamphshire General Asylum, where he spent the rest of his days, suffering periodic lapses of memory and continued bouts of depression, but continuing to write poetry.

Wiley Clements (1928–)

Clements was born in rural Alabama. He lives in Lewisburg, Pennsylvania, in retirement after a long career first as a military journalist, later as a developer of health maintenance organizations (HMOs). He was editor of *The Susquehanna Quarterly* from 1998 to 2002.

Lucille Clifton (1936–)

Clifton was born in Depew, New York, and grew up in Buffalo. Her parents never finished grade school, but they encouraged her academic pursuits. At age sixteen she entered Howard University on a full scholarship, a contemporary of Toni Morrison (Chloe Wofford at the time). After three years studying drama she transferred to Fredonia State Teachers College and began writing poetry and drama. She published her first poetry collection in 1969 after winning a young poets award. By this time she was married and had six children, and with the success of her first book she continued to publish. She taught at the University of California at Santa Cruz, American University, and St. Mary's College of Maryland. Her work has addressed issues of race and oppression, and has also examined her personal struggles with the early deaths of both her husband and mother. She served as poet laureate of Maryland from 1979 to 1982 and taught at Columbia University from 1995 to 1999.

Samuel Taylor Coleridge (1772–1834)

Coleridge was born in Devonshire, the youngest son of a local priest who died when Samuel was nine years old. Coleridge attended Christ's

Hospital School in London and received a scholarship to attend Jesus College, Cambridge. He left school after two years to attempt to join the army, but subsequently returned to Cambridge. Coleridge left school a second time after meeting fellow poet Robert Southey in 1794, with whom he devised a plan to move to America and start a new society. Though the utopian plan dissolved, he married the sister of Southey's wife. Coleridge developed an addiction to opiates while being treated for a variety of physical complaints. He became friends with William Wordsworth and developed an infatuation with his sister-in-law. In 1804 he moved to Malta for two years, then returned to England, where his depression and addiction had impaired his marriage and friendships. In 1816 he sought the help from, and subsequently moved into the household of, Dr. Gilman, who attempted to strictly control and gradually reduce his opiate use. He lived with the Gilmans at Highgate until his death in 1834.

William Collins (1721–1759)

Collins was born in Chichester and attended Queen's College, Oxford. He left for London at a young age, penniless, to try his hand as a writer. He was published, though not extensively. After a trip to France he was placed in an asylum, and following his release he spent the rest of his life in the care of his sister.

Richard David Comstock (birth/death dates unknown; published 1930)

Comstock was a patient at New Jersey State Hospital at Greystone Park. His interests were in horticulture and engineering, though according to his book-long poem, he had little hope of recovering these interests when he was first hospitalized. After several months of hospitalization, he began to write. In 1930 the hospital print shop published his poetry collection, *Rhymes of a Raver*, the inspiration for which he attributed to his fellow "inmates" and to the staff of Greystone Park. Shortly after completing the book, which he described as his "first and last," he was to be discharged "out into the great, new, glorious world of hopeful achievement and endeavor."

William Cowper (1731–1800)

Cowper was born into nobility in Berkhamsted, the son of the Reverend John Cowper and grandson of the chief justice of Chester; his brother served as high chancellor of England. After his mother died at age six, Cowper battled both early eyesight trouble and extreme shyness. Nonetheless, he went on to study law, though he never practiced. Beginning at about age twenty-one he suffered recurrent bouts of depression, and also became acutely aware of recurrent severe depressive episodes in his uncle Ashley Cowper. In the wake of a stressful job interview he made three attempts to kill himself by a variety of means. In 1763 he was admitted to Dr. Nathaniel Cotton's asylum in St. Albans, where he arrived violent and delusional. Depressive symptoms and profound social anxiety were intermixed with evangelical and missionary fervor in a pattern that waxed and waned for the remainder of his life, which was spent either institutionalized or under the care of similarly evangelical families.

Hart Crane (1899–1932)

Crane was born in the suburbs of Cleveland, Ohio. He left high school before graduation and moved to New York City in 1916. For the next seven years he worked odd jobs in New York City and Cleveland, including helping with the candy factory his father owned and writing copy for various retail magazines. He lived a transient life, moving between friends' homes, traveling Europe and Mexico, and occasionally returning to a family retreat on an island off of Cuba. This itinerant lifestyle included love affairs with various men, though he had no stable partners after the age of twenty-five. Most of his poetry was written between 1925 and 1926, but a wealthy patron sponsored the publication of his longest and most famous piece, "The Bridge," in 1930. Crane used alcohol heavily and experienced bouts of depression. The early 1930s were a time of stress for Crane, due to the death of his father and his failure to be productive during a fellowship to write about the Aztec civilization in Mexico. He is thought to have committed suicide in 1932 by jumping off a ship headed back to the U.S. from Mexico, though accident cannot be ruled out.

J. V. (James Vincent) Cunningham (1911–1985)

Cunningham was born in Cumberland, Maryland, and grew up in Billings, Montana. He attended a Jesuit high school and graduated at the age of fifteen but could not proceed further in his education because of the financial situation of his family after his father died. Moving to Denver, Cunningham worked at the Denver Stock Exchange until the 1929 stock market crash, and then began a nomadic work life. He subsequently attended Stanford University, studying with the poet

Yvor Winters. He received his Ph.D. in 1945, subsequently teaching at the University of Chicago, the University of Hawaii, Harvard, the University of Virginia, and Washington University. He was married three times, and he settled in 1953 at Brandeis University, where he remained until his death from heart failure.

Sir John Davies (c. 1565–1618)

Davies began his working life as a scribe in London, eventually settling with a practice in law and entering Parliament. He was recognized as a poet throughout his career by Queen Elizabeth and was knighted solicitor general of Ireland by King James IV in 1603. He later served as attorney general of Ireland, and shortly before his death he was appointed chief justice of England.

Timothy Dekin (1943–2001)

Dekin grew up in Ilion, New York. He taught at Loyola University, Stanford University, and Northwestern University. His poetry addresses not only his love of the outdoors and fishing, but also his difficult childhood and persistent battle with alcoholism. He died at the age of fifty-eight, a year before his first poetry collection was published.

Emily Dickinson (1830–1886)

Born in Amherst, Massachusetts, Dickinson received most of her education in her Puritan household, remaining close to her family for the entirety of her life. She attended Amherst Academy and Mount Holyoke, though she left for periods because of homesickness. She lived with her parents thereafter. She wrote over one thousand poems but published only seven in her lifetime, with support from Thomas Wentworth Higginson and Helen Hunt Jackson. Her shy and isolated lifestyle became more extreme during her thirties, and this isolation has prompted much speculation about emotional problems. Most of the details of her life remain unknown. Her sister found the majority of her poetry bound in her bureau after Emily's death, though on Dickinson's own request all her letters were burned.

Sydney Dobell (1824–1874)

Dobell was born in Cranbrook, Kent, into a family of means and of political and religious radicalism. He married and maintained both an active literary career and an extensive involvement in his family's wine business. Dobell developed a strong interest in the reunification struggles of Italy and published a commercially successful, long, politically oriented poem, "The Roman," under the pseudonym Sydney Yendys. However, his second major lengthy work, "Balder," took as its focus the life of the mind of a poet, Balder, who, "egoistic, self-contained, and sophistical, imperfect in morality, and destitute of organized religion" (Dobell's description), was widely reviled by the public. Dobell was attacked by a variety of literary figures including W. E. Aytoun, who described Dobell as leading the "Spasmodic School of Poetry." Dobell continued to publish verse and an occasional critical piece, though he never regained the popular acclaim of the pre-Balder days. He and his wife returned to Italy, where he suffered a traumatic brain injury from a fall and developed epilepsy. He did not write during the last years of his life.

Ernest Dowson (1867–1900)

Dowson was born in Kent, though his father moved the family to France shortly after Ernest was born. He went on to attend Queen's College, Oxford, in 1886, but left after a year without a degree. He became a convert to Roman Catholicism in 1891, the same year he fell in unrequited love with a twelve-year-old girl who was to become the subject of many of his poems. He moved to London in 1894 in the aftermath of his father's death under questionable conditions and his mother's subsequent suicide. In London he became a literary colleague of Oscar Wilde, Aubrey Beardsley, and W. B. Yeats, and a member of the Rhymers' Club. He subsequently moved to Paris and then to Ireland. He lived an extravagant lifestyle, using alcohol heavily and spending money carelessly. By 1899 Dowson had returned to London in poverty, likely sick with tuberculosis, and died at age thirty-two.

William Dunbar (1460–1513)

Dunbar was born in Salton, East Lothian, in Scotland. Little is known about his life, though it is thought that he went to St. Andrews University. Records indicate that between 1500 and 1513 he received a salary from James IV. He served in James's court, which was the setting for most of his poetry. In 1504 he was ordained as a priest, and then appointed court chaplain, with records also describing his participation in some of the court's legal cases. His last recorded presence in James's court comes from 1513, shortly before the battle of Flodden, in which the king and many members of his house were killed.

Robert Duncan (1919–1988)

Duncan was born in Oakland, California, with the given name of Edward Howard Duncan. When his mother died in childbirth, his father was forced for financial reasons to put him up for adoption, and the architect who adopted him renamed him Robert Edward Symmes. His adoptive family was extremely spiritual, and brought him up in the same fashion. Despite an early injury that resulted in permanent double vision, Duncan was an avid reader and in 1936 attended the University of California at Berkeley for two years, during which time his first poems were published. He moved to Woodstock, New York, after a failed relationship with one of his male teachers. He was drafted and sent to San Antonio, then discharged because of, officially, a psychological disturbance; he later recounted that the underlying reason was his homosexuality. In 1943 he married a woman, though they were divorced shortly afterward. In 1945 he returned to San Francisco and in 1948 to Berkeley to study for two more years. In 1951 he met the painter Jess Collins, with whom he settled in San Francisco. He died of kidney disease.

Robert Fergusson (1750–1774)

Fergusson was born in Edinburgh. Due to early sickness he started schooling late, but entered St. Andrews University at the young age of fourteen. The poet William Wilkie took a great liking to Fergusson at St. Andrews. However, Fergusson left school in 1768 without a diploma (after participating in student riots) and to attend to his family after his father's death. Returning home, he worked copying documents in the local commissary office, and gained a reputation in Edinburgh theater. In 1771 his first three poems were published anonymously in *Ruddiman's Magazine*, which afterward sponsored his writing. In 1774 he left work, manifesting obsessive religious behavior that included burning his own writings; some have speculated that this behavior change was due to syphilis, others, to depression. In 1774, after a serious head injury due to falling down stairs, he became delusional and was sent to Edinburgh's Bedlam. He died there a year later, most likely of complications from the injury.

Anne Finch, Countess of Winchilsea (1661–1720)

Finch was born into a wealthy family and received an education unusually comprehensive for women of her time. She married early and became the Countess of Winchilsea. She was encouraged in her writing throughout her life by her husband, as well as by her friends Alexander Pope and Jonathan Swift. She wrote candidly about the political and religious turmoil plaguing England, but also about her personal struggles with periods of depression, a condition that worsened toward the end of her life.

John Fletcher (1579–1625)

As son of the bishop of Bristol, Worcester, and London, Fletcher grew up studying the classics, and went on to a literary career. He never married and died of the plague in London at age forty-six. Copublication and multiple attribution of authorship were not uncommon at this time; for instance, there is evidence that Shakespeare (q.v.) may have collaborated with Fletcher and Thomas Middleton (q.v.), among others, on some of his plays. "Melancholy" has been attributed both to Fletcher and to Thomas Middleton. Fletcher's literary information is also often coupled with that of his close friend and frequent coauthor, Francis Beaumont.

Allen Ginsberg (1926–1997)

Ginsberg was born to a middle-class family in Newark, New Jersey, and grew up in Paterson. In 1943 he entered Columbia University. During his time there he met the nucleus of writers who would become the "Beat" movement, including William S. Burrows and Jack Kerouac. He was expelled from Columbia but returned for graduate studies. In 1949 he was implicated in storing stolen goods, pled insanity, and was sent to the New York State Psychiatric Institute (NYSPI), where he stayed for eight months. During this time he met Carl Solomon (q.v.), to whom he later dedicated "Howl." Their meeting at NYPSI has become an iconic moment in the history of American letters, with Solomon reportedly greeting Ginsberg saying, "I'm Kirilov" (from Dostoyevsky's *The Possessed*), and Ginsberg responding, "I'm Myshkin" (from *The Idiot*). Prior to his stay in NYSPI, Ginsberg had been in psychoanalysis, and in 1948 he reported hearing the voice of Blake (q.v.), or God, when reading Blake's poetry. In 1954 Ginsberg moved to San Francisco and soon published "Howl," which began his literary reputation—enhanced by obscenity charges and arrest of the poem's publisher, the poet Lawrence Ferlinghetti. Heavy use of drugs for consciousness-raising or recreation was part of the Beat culture, and Ginsberg was no exception among its members. However, in 1962 he traveled to India, eschewed drugs for meditation, and became a disciple of the Tibetan Buddhist abbot Chögyam Trungpa Rinpoche. In 1974 Ginsberg began a branch of Trungpa's Naropa Institute in Boulder, Colorado, which he named the Jack Kerouac School of Disembodied Poetics. After a long and highly visible life in American letters, politics, and social change, Ginsberg died of cardiovascular causes and liver cancer in 1997.

Matthew Green (1696–1737)
Green was born in England and was raised in a Nonconformist household. He worked as a clerk and began writing without intentions of publication. His most famous piece, "The Spleen," may have merely been a letter of advice to his close friend Mr. Cuthbert Jackson. He lived at Nag's Head Court, Gracechurch Street, and died there, unmarried, at the age of forty-one.

Fulke Greville (1554–1628)
Greville was born into nobility in Beauchamp Court, Warwickshire. He was educated at Shrewsbury School and then Jesus College, Cambridge, where he became friends with the poet Sir Philip Sidney. In 1577 he entered the court of Elizabeth I with Sidney. He held many titles, including secretary of the principality of Wales, Knight of the Bath, treasurer of the Navy, and chancellor of the exchequer. He was named Lord Brooke by James I. Only two of his poems were published in his lifetime. Greville was killed in 1628 by one of his servants, whom he had not included in his will, and the servant then killed himself.

Aimee Grunberger (1951–1995)
Grunberger was born in Stamford, Connecticut. She attended Brown University, graduating with honors in 1975 and subsequently studying clinical psychology at the University of Massachusetts. She received her master's degree from Naropa Institute (see Ginsberg entry), where she returned later to teach in summer writing programs. She worked as a psychotherapist in Providence, Rhode Island, at the Department of Veterans Affairs Medical Center. In 1991 she moved with her husband and twin sons to Boulder, Colorado, where she died of cancer at the age of forty-four.

Ivor Gurney (1890–1937)
Gurney was born in Gloucester near the Cotswolds and was encouraged in literary and musical pursuits by his godfather. In 1911 he entered the

Royal College of Music in London on a scholarship; while there he was considered extremely talented but unpredictable. In 1912 he became depressed and returned to Gloucestershire. In 1914 he volunteered for military service and was turned down because of poor eyesight, but in 1915 he enlisted successfully. He served as a private in the trenches in France. During this time a fellow soldier lent him an anthology by Robert Bridges (q.v.), and Gurney began to write poetry intensely, with his first book published in 1917. Shortly thereafter he was wounded and gassed, and was hospitalized. In 1918 he was discharged with "deferred shell shock." From 1919 to 1922 Gurney worked a variety of jobs, returned briefly to the Royal College to study music under Ralph Vaughan Williams, and published a second volume of poetry and a number of musical pieces. In 1922 he began to act bizarrely, suffering paranoid delusions and repeatedly going to the police, family, and friends to ask for a gun to shoot himself. In 1922 his family committed him to Barnswood House, a private asylum in Gloucester. Later that year he was transferred to the City of London Mental Hospital, where he spent the rest of his life, continuing to write poetry and music. A third volume of his poems was published in 1954, and additional poems have been published in several collections since the 1990s.

Thomas Hardy (1840–1928)

Hardy was born and home-schooled in Dorset by his middle-class working parents. He apprenticed with an architect at the age of sixteen, while studying poetry and classics on his own. Unsuccessful in publishing poetry initially, he wrote novels instead. His novels were met at first with mixed reviews and then with substantial success despite their controversial subject matter, which called to question traditional Victorian values. He married in 1874, and in the 1890s, after becoming well known for fifteen novels and fifty short stories, he returned to poetry. The Hardys' marriage had been difficult, but when his wife died in 1912, he wrote a substantial amount of poetry about their relationship. In 1914 he married his much younger secretary, with whom he lived and worked until his death at age eighty-eight in Dorset.

Jim Harrison (1937–)

Harrison was born in northern Michigan and received his bachelor's and master's degrees from Michigan State University. He taught English at the State University of New York at Stony Brook. In addition to poetry, he has written nonfiction, novels, and novellas. Two of his novellas, *Legends of the Fall* and *Revenge*, have been made into movies. He now lives in nothern Michigan.

William Harrison (1685–1713)

Little is known about Harrison's life. According to his friend Edward Young (q.v), he was a fellow at New College, Oxford. We are told this in a footnote at the end of Young's very long "Epistle to the Right Honorable George, Lord Lansdowne," which concludes with a lament of Harrison's untimely death. We know from Jonathon Swift's journals and letters that Swift arranged for Harrison to become editor of *The Tatler*, a many-lived newspaper of literary and social issues. Swift also arranged for Harrison to take a position as secretary to the embassy at Utrecht. Shortly after returning to England, Harrison died at age twenty-eight.

Anthony Hecht (1923–2004)

Hecht was born in New York City and grew up on the Upper East Side. He enrolled in Bard College at the age of seventeen, where he began to write poetry. When World War II broke out, Hecht joined the U.S. Army and served in Europe and Japan. Upon his return he studied at Kenyon College under John Crowe Ransom, received his master's degree at Columbia University, and subsequently became a professor at Kenyon. He also taught at Smith College, Bard College, Columbia University, Towson State University, the University of Rochester, Georgetown, Washington University, Yale, and Harvard. He was divorced in 1961 from his first wife, by whom he had two children, and he remarried in 1971. He died at home with his second wife and his son in Washington, DC, of non-Hodgkin's lymphoma.

George Herbert (1593–1633)

Herbert was born in Montgomery, Wales, to an upper-class family. His father died when he was three, but his mother, who was a close acquaintance of the poet John Donne, ensured that all of her ten children received a proper education. Herbert attended Westminster School and subsequently received a scholarship to Trinity College, Cambridge. He was elected fellow of the college, and in 1620 was named public orator of the University. Herbert was chosen to serve in the royal court but instead stepped down from his position as orator in order to pursue a career in the clergy. He married in 1629. Herbert often endured long periods of fasting and contemplation, and had a reputation for self-sacrifice and benevolence. His poetry remained unpublished until the year of his death of tuberculosis at the age of forty.

Robert Herrick (1591–1674)

Herrick was born in Cheapside, London, into a wealthy family of goldsmiths. His father died during Robert's first year from a fatal fall out of a window, following the writing of his will. Robert attended St. John's College and Trinity College, Cambridge. After graduating in 1620, Herrick joined a group of London poets known as "Sons of Ben," associated with the poet Ben Jonson, before eventually taking a position that required him to move to the countryside as dean prior of Devonshire. He fathered a child but never married. With the rise of the Commonwealth, Herrick lost his position temporarily and worked in London, writing extensively until 1662. He regained his position as dean prior and served in that capacity until his death in 1674.

Thomas Hoccleve (c. 1368–c. 1426)

Hoccleve was a younger acquaintance of Chaucer, and served as a clerk at the office of the Privy Seal at Westminster where Chaucer was clerk of works. Records as early as 1407 show Hoccleve's increasing anxiety about his financial straits, despite his having a stable job. About 1416 he suffered some sort of breakdown that took five years to resolve. "The Complaint" is his first work after this period, and describes his attempts to reintegrate into society. The themes that emerge from this work are familiar to modern readers, including feelings of alienation from and stigmatization by his peers. In some aspects his unusually personal poem anticipates the confessional poets of the 1950s and 1960s.

Jeff Holt (1971–)

Holt is a licensed professional counselor who has worked with severely mentally ill adults, adolescents, and children. He currently works for a managed behavioral health care company and lives with his wife, Sarena, in Plano, Texas. Holt's work has appeared in the anthology *Sonnets: 150 Contemporary Sonnets*, edited by William Baer, and in a variety of literary journals including *The Formalist, The Texas Review, Measure, The Evansville Review, Rattapallax, Iambs & Trochees, Pivot, Cumberland Poetry Review*, and *Sparrow*.

Gerard Manley Hopkins (1844–1889)

Hopkins was born in Stratford, Essex, and was educated at Oxford, where he and Robert Bridges (q.v.) became friends and literary companions. After converting to Catholicism under the influence of John Henry Newman, he entered the Jesuit order. When he became a Jesuit he burned the poetry he had written, thinking it unseemly for a priest to have written secular verse. With permission of his superiors, he published "The Wreck of the Deutschland" about the death of a group of nuns in a shipwreck, but he wrote little for publication thereafter. He was appointed professor of classics at University College in Dublin. He experienced a sense of exile in Ireland both physically and spiritually. Out of this period came his "terrible sonnets." He died at the age of forty-four, unrecognized as a poet. His poetry was not published until 1918 when his friend Bridges compiled his works.

Richard Hugo (1923–1982)

Hugo was born near Seattle, Washington. His father left his mother after his birth, and two years later his mother placed him in the care of her parents, who raised him in modest circumstances. He attended public school during the Great Depression, and occupied himself with books, baseball, and fishing. In 1942 he entered the Army Air Corps, serving for two years in Italy as a bomber pilot. With the GI Bill he was able to attend the University of Washington, where he studied under Theodore Roethke (q.v.). In 1952 he married and started a thirteen-year career as a technical writer at Boeing aircraft company. In 1963 he returned to Italy with his wife, though after a year they were divorced. Hugo subsequently taught at the University of Montana, and he remarried in 1975. He also taught briefly at the University of Iowa and the University of Washington, and served as editor of the Yale Younger Poet Series. Hugo died of leukemia.

Mark Jarman (1952–)

Jarman was born in Mount Sterling, Kentucky, and grew up in California and Scotland, where his father served as a minister. He graduated in 1974 from the University of California at Santa Cruz, having previously won a poetry award. He attended the Iowa Writers' Workshop and earned his MFA from the University of Iowa, working with Donald Justice (q.v.), Sandra McPherson, and Charles Wright. Jarman subsequently taught at Indiana State University, the University of California at Irvine, Murray State University in Kentucky, and, most recently, Vanderbilt University as a professor of English. In addition to extensive poetry and critical work, he is the editor of the journal *The Reaper*. He lives in Nashville, Tennessee, with his wife and two daughters.

Randall Jarrell (1914–1965)

Jarrell was born in Nashville, Tennessee, though he spent much of his youth in Los Angeles. He attended Vanderbilt University and was mentored by Robert Penn Warren, John Crow Ransom, and Allen Tate (q.v.). He followed Ransom to Kenyon in 1937 and taught there for two years. At Kenyon he roomed briefly with Robert Lowell (q.v.), and then moved to teach at the University of Texas. He married and published his first poems in 1940, and from 1942 to 1946 served in the Army Air Force. He subsequently worked as literary editor for *The Nation* for a year, and went on to teach at Sarah Lawrence College and then at the University of North Carolina. Depression led to a suicide attempt and subsequent psychiatric admission in North Carolina. He died shortly after discharge, hit by a car while walking along a road in the early evening. Suicide was openly suspected, but never confirmed.

Donald Justice (1925–2004)

Justice was born in Miami, Florida, and enrolled in the University of Miami to study music. He changed his area of study to English, and after working for a short while in New York, received an MA at the University of North Carolina in 1947. He married Jean Ross, a classmate and fellow writer, the same year. He began to teach at the University of Miami, but after a year he enrolled in a Ph.D. program at Stanford University. He then returned to teach in Miami until 1952. He subsequently enrolled in the Iowa Writers' Workshop and received his Ph.D. from the University of Iowa. He taught at the Workshop for ten years. His first collection was published in 1960, and he held teaching jobs at Syracuse University, the University of California at Irvine, and the University of Florida. In 1991 he wrote a libretto for an opera, and from 1992 lived in Iowa City with his wife and son.

John Keats (1795–1821)

Born in a stable in Moorfields, London, Keats survived a troubled childhood. His father was not well-off and died in an accident when Keats was nine, and his mother died of tuberculosis only six years later.

At fifteen years of age he left school and trained with a surgeon but never practiced medicine. At nineteen he left for London and worked as an apothecary the following year. With the assistance of his friends Leigh Hunt, Percy Shelley (q.v.), and William Wordsworth, Keats began publishing. He fell in love with Fanny Brawne in 1818, and the two were briefly engaged before he died, at age twenty-six, of tuberculosis. Some sources maintain that Keats suffered one or more bouts of venereal disease in his lifetime, as he was treated on several occasions with mercury, a common remedy for such infections.

Weldon Kees (1914–1955)

Kees was born in Beatrice, Nebraska, and participated enthusiastically in art, music, and writing from a young age. Despite the Great Depression, he was able to attend the University of Nebraska and graduated in 1935, having already published some works of fiction in local magazines. He began working for the Federal Writers' Project in Lincoln, but left in 1937 for Denver, where he got married and began a job as a librarian. In 1943 he moved to New York City, where he began to publish extensively, often in *Time* magazine, the *New York Times*, and the *New Yorker*. He also took up painting in New York, with several gallery showings, including representation at the 1950 Whitney Annual. In 1950 Kees left New York City for San Francisco, where he wrote poetry, painted, wrote jazz, and played piano for a number of groups. He worked on films and documentaries, though his life grew complicated with his wife's increasing alcoholism and psychiatric difficulties. They divorced in 1954 and Kees spoke often of the need for drastic change in his life, with plans possibly to leave America. In the summer of 1955 his car was discovered with the keys inside parked by the Golden Gate Bridge. His whereabouts thereafter were never established, and his body was never found.

Henry Kendall (1839–1882)

Kendall was born to poor but educated parents on a small farm in Kirmington, New South Wales, Australia. After his father's death when Henry was thirteen, Kendall lived with relatives and worked aboard his uncle's ship until 1857 when he moved to Sydney. He worked delivery jobs until attaining a position as a clerk, at which point he began submitting his poems to magazines and journals. He was published and attracted the attention of some wealthy benefactors. In 1868, with a secure job in the government, he married Charlotte Rutter, whom he met after one of his lectures at the Sydney School of the Arts. He spent two years battling depression and difficulty with alcohol, seeking refuge with a family of timber workers in Gosford. In 1880 he attained a civil service job as inspector of Forests, but he died of tuberculosis in 1882.

Jane Kenyon (1947–1995)

Kenyon was born in Ann Arbor, Michigan. She attended the University of Michigan, where she met her future husband, English professor and poet Donald Hall. In 1972 after her graduation, the couple moved to a farm in Wilmont, New Hampshire, where they published extensively. Kenyon was quite public regarding her difficulties with depression, discussing it both in her poetry and in documentaries and interviews. She was diagnosed with leukemia, continuing to serve as poet laureate for the state of New Hampshire until her death. The couple's struggle with her illness and death are the subject of Hall's volume of poems *Without*.

Yusef Komunyakaa (1947–)

Komunyakaa was born in Bogalusa, Louisiana, and spent much of his youth immersed in the music scene of New Orleans. After attending public high school in Bogalusa, he interrupted his education to join the U.S. Army in Vietnam, where he wrote for and edited the war newspaper *The Southern Cross*. Upon his return he entered the University of Colorado, where he began to write poetry. He received his master's degree from Colorado State University and MFA at the University of California at Irvine. He returned to Louisiana to teach at the University of New Orleans, and subsequently taught at Indiana University while publishing extensively. He currently teaches at Princeton University.

Stanley Kunitz (1905–2006)

Kunitz was born in Worcester, Massachusetts. His father had committed suicide shortly before Stanley's birth, after the family's dress business went bankrupt. Kunitz grew attached to a stepfather, who died when Kunitz was fourteen. His mother worked hard to raise her children while paying off debts. Kunitz received a scholarship to Harvard, where he also received his master's degree. He moved to New York in 1927 and started work as a journalist. The following year his poetry began to be published in various magazines, including *The Nation*. When World War II broke out, Kunitz was denied status as a conscientious objector and fought with the U.S. Army for three years.

Upon his return in 1946 he taught at Bennington College, and later held positions at Columbia, Yale, Rutgers, Princeton, and the University of Washington. He also helped establish the Fine Arts Work Center in Provincetown, Massachusetts, and the Poets House in New York City. In 2000 he served as poet laureate of the United States. He married three times and had one daughter. He died at the age of 100.

Philip Larkin (1922–1985)
Larkin was born in Coventry, Warwickshire. His family life was stressful, with his mother chronically unhappy and his father the Coventry treasurer and reputedly a Nazi sympathizer. Larkin attended King Henry VIII School in Coventry, where he had a difficult time socially due to poor eyesight and a speech impediment. However, he wrote for the school magazine, and in 1940 went on to study English at St. John's College, Oxford. Larkin was not drafted because of his eyesight, and was also unable to get a job in the civil service when he graduated. He settled for work in Shropshire as a librarian, a profession he would maintain for the majority of his life. He subsequently served as librarian at the university libraries at Leicester and at Belfast, and finally at the Brynmor Jones Library at the University of Hull. After a long series of liaisons, in 1974 he moved in with his lover, Monica Jones. He died of throat cancer.

Michael Lauchlan (1954–)
Lauchlan has lived in and around Detroit for his entire life and has devoted much of his energy to a variety of community groups in roles as various as builder, organizer, and grant-writer. His most recent chapbook is *Sudden Parade* from Riverside Press. His poems have appeared in *New England Review*, *Virginia Quarterly Review*, *Victoria Park*, the *North American Review*, and in *Abandoned Automobile*, an anthology of Detroit poetry from Wayne State University Press. Since completing his MFA from Warren Wilson College in 1991, Lauchlan reports that he has been teaching English, coaching baseball, and enjoying his family.

Thomas Lodge (c. 1557–1625)
Lodge was the son of the lord mayor of London and studied at Merchant Taylors School and then Trinity College, Oxford, originally preparing for a law career. Instead he began writing plays and poetry, as well as

publishing pamphlets sufficiently controversial to have been banned. He traveled with the poet Thomas Cavendish to South America, lost his family's inheritance, and fell into debt later in life. Subsequently he trained as a physician at Avignon and Oxford and practiced as a physician in London after 1596. He married twice and converted to Roman Catholicism upon his second marriage.

Robert Lowell (1917–1977)

Lowell's patrician family included the poets James Russell Lowell and Amy Lowell. He left Harvard College after two years, and with encouragement from Allen Tate (q.v.) finished his undergraduate studies at Kenyon College under the mentorship of John Crown Ransom. His poetry ranged widely, but, unusual for that time, much of his poetry dealt explicitly with personal circumstances that deeply affected him. These included his conversion to Catholicism, his failed marriage to fellow writer Jean Stafford, and his experiences in jail as a conscientious objector during World War II. However, among the most striking and innovative of these "confessional" themes was the explicit incorporation of his struggles with manic-depression and alcohol abuse, including his experiences during multiple psychiatric hospitalizations.

Kelly Ann Malone (1963–)

Malone was born and raised in Southern California. She has been writing since she was around twelve years old. She reports that some of her poetic influences are Ogden Nash, Edna St. Vincent Millay (q.v.), Sara Teasdale, Emily Dickinson (q.v.), Billy Collins, and Dorothy Parker (q.v.).

Thomas Middleton (1580–1627)

Middleton was born in London into a bricklayer's family. His father died when Middleton was six years old, and his mother remarried within a year afterward. His childhood was one of financial and emotional instability. He attended Queen's College, Oxford, but left in 1601 due to family issues and returned to London. He began writing in London, where he could be paid for his plays, and worked alongside Philip Henslowe at the Rose Theatre. By 1613 he was writing for the lord mayor, and in 1620 he was deemed city chronologer for London. In 1623 he had a son, though record of marriage has not been found. He coauthored much of his work with Thomas Dekker during this period. Copublication and multiple attribution of authorship were not uncommon at this time. "Melancholy" has been attributed to both Middleton and John Fletcher (q.v.).

Edna St. Vincent Millay (1892–1950)

Millay was born in Rockland, Maine. Her mother, who divorced her father when Edna was eight, worked as a single mother. Millay received a scholarship to Vassar after winning an award in a poetry contest. As an undergraduate she wrote for numerous magazines and journals while also acting and writing plays. She moved to Greenwich Village after college and developed an extensive circle of literary and theatrical peers. Paid as a writer by *Vanity Fair*, Millay was able to travel Europe in 1920, and in 1923 she became the first woman to receive the Pulitzer Prize. Also in that year she married Eugen Jan Boissenvain, though she was openly bisexual. In 1928 Millay suffered the loss of her close friend, poet Elinor Wylie, followed by the death of her mother and father a few years later. In the aftermath of these deaths, she suffered prolonged depression, depending heavily on her husband and unable to write from 1944 to 1945. Both she and Boissenvain struggled with alcoholism. Millay died in 1950 of a heart attack on her farm in the Berkshires.

John Milton (1608–1674)

Milton was born in Cheapside, London, where he was raised in a religious household and was tutored in the classics. He attended St. Paul's School, followed by Christ's College, Cambridge. In Cambridge, to his father's dismay, he pursued poetry and playwriting instead of joining the ministry. In 1638 he traveled Europe, where he met a number of influential people, including Galileo, Hugo Grotius, and Giovanni Batista. He eventually returned to London, then in political turmoil, and sided with Cromwell against Charles I. He married a much younger Mary Powell. They separated for three years, and she returned to him in 1645, the year as his first poems were published. In 1652 Milton lost his eyesight, his wife died after childbirth, and shortly thereafter his only son died. He remarried twice, was arrested briefly for his political writing when Charles II came to power, and finished his life removed from politics, during which time he wrote *Paradise Lost*.

Thomas Mozeen (birth/death dates unknown; published 1768)

Mozeen was born in England of French ancestry. Little is known about his life except that he worked as a comic actor and singer on stages in Dublin, wrote a book detailing the nomadic life of an actor, and published essays in London around 1762. He was known to stay with his friend the Earl of Kilruddery for summers at the Loughlinstown Inn in County Wicklow, where he wrote about the hunting and drinking habits of the various visiting nobility.

Les Murray (1938–)

Murray was born in the rural town of Nabiac, New South Wales, Australia, where his parents owned a dairy farm. The family was often on the brink of poverty and eventually lost their farm. Murray entered the University of Sydney in 1957. During his time there he worked on undergraduate literary publications and converted to Roman Catholicism. Murray left Sydney after three years and became a translator at the Australian National University at Canberra. In 1965 he published his first collection of poetry, and shortly thereafter he left Australia to travel to Europe for a year. He returned to the University of Sydney and graduated in 1969, subsequently working as a freelance writer, critic, and editor for multiple Sydney publications. In 1988 he left Sydney to return to farm life and to write in New South Wales. His book-length verse narrative, *Fredy Neptune*, relates the adventures of a young Australian of German descent during and after World War I. Fredy develops an unexplained inability to feel physical pain after witnessing a gang of Turks burning Armenian women to death in Istanbul. The book chronicles Fredy's eventual psychosomatic and spiritual recovery.

Howard Nemerov (1920–1991)

Nemerov was born in New York City into an accomplished family. His father was the head of a fashion store, and his sister was the well-known photographer Diane Arbus, who committed suicide in 1940. Nemerov attended Fieldston School and then Harvard, graduating in 1941. From 1941 to 1945 Nemerov fought in World War II, flying with the U.S. Army Air Corps. He married during this time and returned with his wife to New York City. Within a year he had a son, and his first book of poetry was published. His teaching career began in 1946 at Hamilton College, followed by teaching at Bennington College, then Brandeis University, and finally Washington University in St. Louis, where he taught from 1969 until his death. In 1988 he was named U.S. poet laureate.

Ned O'Gorman (1929–)

O'Gorman was born in New York City and grew up between Southport, Connecticut, and Bradford, Vermont. He attended Saint Michael's

College in Vermont and then entered graduate studies at Columbia University. He worked as editor of the magazine *Jubilee* between 1962 and 1965, and then worked in South America. He returned to New York City to teach and held positions at Brooklyn College, the New School for Social Research, and Manhattan College. In 1966 he founded the Children's Storefront School in Harlem, working as headmaster for thirty-two years. In 1998 he founded the Ricardo O'Gorman Garden and School, named after his son who died at the age of twenty-six.

Sharon Olds (1942–)

Olds was born in San Francisco. Her father suffered from difficulties with alcohol, contributing to a complex relationship with Olds that she has explored extensively in her poetry. She attended Stanford and then Columbia University where she received her Ph.D. in English, subsequently settling in New York City. She began publishing poetry when she was thirty-seven, her first collection examining of the complexity of family relationships. By 1988 she had won numerous awards and was named poet laureate for New York State. She currently teaches at the New York University Graduate Creative Writing Program, including staffing NYU's writing outreach program at Goldwater Hospital, a physical rehabilitation center.

Charles d'Orleans (1394–1465)

Charles was the nephew of the French king Charles VI. At age twelve he was married to his cousin Isabelle, and the following year his father was murdered by the Duke of Burgundy. His mother died in 1408, and at fourteen he was named Duke of Orleans. In 1415 he was captured by the English during hostilities and was held prisoner for twenty-five years, during which time he wrote most of his poetry. In 1447 he left for Italy to claim the family estate, where he lived until the age of sixty-nine with his daughter and son, who would later become King Louis XII.

Wilfred Owen (1893–1918)

Owen was born in Shropshire where his father worked at the railroad station. He studied at Shrewsbury Technical School and sought a scholarship to the University of London. When he did not receive the scholarship, Owen took it upon himself to study with the vicar of Dunsden in Oxfordshire, where he began to experiment with poetry.

Owen subsequently taught in Bordeaux in 1913 at the Berlitz School of Languages. After a year he began to work as a private tutor, and in 1915 he enlisted in the London Regiment and became a lieutenant. In 1917 he entered Craiglockhart War Hospital for Nervous Disorders, after surviving severe shelling in battle. There he met Siegfried Sassoon (q.v.) and through Sassoon was introduced to Robert Ross and Robert Graves. In 1918 Owen was presented with a Military Cross for bravery. He was killed in battle a month later at age twenty-five.

Dorothy Parker (1893–1967)
Parker was born in West End, New Jersey. Her mother died when she was very young, and she had difficulties with her father, her step-mother, and at her Catholic convent school. In 1912 after her father died she moved to Greenwich Village, New York City, initially earning a living playing piano. After submitting a poem to *Vanity Fair*, she was accepted first as a caption writer and then as a critic for the magazine and subsequently for the *New Yorker*. She and several other writers came together as the "Algonquin Round Table," named for the hotel bar at which they regularly met. She was married and divorced, and in 1922 she published her first book. Parker remarried and moved to Beverly Hills, where she began writing screenplays. She battled depression and alcohol throughout her life, including suicide attempts in 1923 and 1925.

Stuart Z. Perkoff (1930–1974)
Perkoff was born in St. Louis. He settled in Venice, California, and eventually became associated with the Beat movement. By the 1960s he had developed an addiction to heroin and was jailed in 1968, serving a prison term of three years. He then started a business selling books in San Francisco and was married twice, his second wife dying of a drug overdose. He returned to Venice in 1973 to start a new writing project, but he died of cancer the following year.

Sylvia Plath (1932–1963)
Plath was born in Boston and lived her early years in Winthrop, Massachusetts. Her father was a professor at Boston University and an expert on bees; he died when Plath was eight years old. Plath's mother moved the family to Wellesley, where she took a job as a teacher. Plath wrote poetry from a very young age, winning local contests and selling her

poems to magazines such as *Seventeen*. She attended Smith College, where she won a college fiction contest sponsored by *Mademoiselle* and sold three poems to *Harper's*. She suffered debilitating depression, including two suicide attempts and psychiatric hospitalization. By age twenty-three she had received electroconvulsive (shock) treatments and insulin coma therapy. However, after a six-month recovery period, Plath returned to school and graduated summa cum laude in 1955. In 1955, on a Fulbright fellowship, she attended Newnham College, Cambridge, where she met and married the English poet Ted Hughes. They returned together to the United States the following year, living in Boston where Plath taught at Smith and studied with Robert Lowell (q.v.). In 1959 Plath and Hughes returned to Britain, moving to Devon to raise their two children. In 1962 they separated and Plath took her children to London, where she began working for the British Broadcasting Corporation while writing her only novel. Two weeks after *The Bell Jar* was published, Plath committed suicide by asphyxiation in her London apartment. She was posthumously awarded the Pulitzer Prize in 1982 for her *Collected Poems*.

A. Mary F. Robinson (1857–1944)

Robinson was born in Leamington, Warwickshire. Her father was a well-known architect, and her childhood was spent in the company of a variety of London artists. She attended preparatory schools in Brussels and Italy and subsequently matriculated at University College London. After graduation she traveled with her close and lifelong confidante Vernon Lee, to whom she would dedicate much of her work. She married in 1888 but was widowed six years later. She remarried and was widowed again two years into that marriage. Robinson wrote for the remainder of her career as Madame Mary Duclaux. She published extensively, both poetry and biography, until her death in France at the age of eighty-seven.

Theodore Roethke (1908–1963)

Roethke was born and raised in Saginaw, Michigan, where his parents ran a large nursery. He attended the University of Michigan, the first in his family to go to college, and graduated with highest honors in 1929. Although at first intending to enter law school, Roethke took English graduate classes at Harvard and subsequently earned his master's degree at the University of Michigan. In 1931 he began teaching at Lafayette College and at the same time developed a friendship with poet Stanley Kunitz (q.v.). Roethke left Lafayette for Michigan State College, where he suffered a depressive episode and was briefly hospitalized. Roethke had a number of subsequent episodes of mania and depression and was hospitalized several times for manic-depressive disorder. Nonetheless, he continued an active teaching career at Pennsylvania State University and then at Bennington College. He left Bennington in 1945 and was subsequently admitted to a hospital in Albany where he received electroconvulsive (shock) treatments. He was sent home to recover under his family's care in Saginaw. In 1947 he resumed teaching and subsequently joined the faculty of the University of Washington, marrying a former Bennington student in 1953. The university was notably supportive of Roethke in his battles with manic-depressive disorder, and he remained on faculty until the year before his death. He died of a heart attack while swimming.

Joseph S. Salemi (1948–)

Salemi teaches in the Department of Humanities at New York University and in the Classics Department of Hunter College. His work has appeared in more than one hundred journals and literary magazines in the United States and in Britain.

Siegfried Sassoon (1886–1967)

Sassoon was born in Weirleigh, Kent, to wealthy parents. They were separated when he was five years old, and his father died of tuberculosis shortly thereafter. Sassoon attended Marlborough College and Clare College, Cambridge, but left after two years. By 1912 Sassoon had privately published nine of his own collections of poetry, and in 1915 he entered World War I as a Royal Welch Fusilier. By the following year Sassoon had lost his younger brother and closest friend in the war and became frustrated with the cause. He began to act recklessly on the battlefield, earning a Military Cross as well as the nickname "Mad Jack." He met Robert Graves, who prevented Sassoon from being prosecuted after throwing his Military Cross into a river. Graves convinced the army that Sassoon needed some time to recover in Craiglockhart War Hospital for Nervous Disorders. While at Craiglockhart, Sassoon wrote prolifically and met the poet Wilfred Owen (q.v.). At age forty-three he married and had a son, but his lovers and companions were primarily men. He converted to Catholicism in 1957 and died in Heytesbury, Wiltshire.

James Schuyler (1923–1991)
Schuyler was born in Chicago and spent two years with the U.S. Navy during World War II. In 1947 he studied in Florence and with W. H. Auden, and upon his return to New York City, was hospitalized in the Westchester Division of New York Hospital, formerly Bloomingdale Asylum. It was the first of a number of hospitalizations in a life complicated by psychiatric symptoms, drugs, and alcohol. A member of the "New York School," much of his work was inspired by the abstract expressionist movement in painting. He worked at the Museum of Modern Art, and was also influenced by the work of his lover, Fairfield Porter. He lived with and depended on Porter's family for over a decade. Schuyler became increasingly reclusive and ill late in life. His poems in this anthology are selected from his series of "Payne Whitney Poems," written while he was hospitalized at that psychiatric facility.

Delmore Schwartz (1913–1966)
Schwartz was born in Brooklyn to immigrant parents; his father became quite wealthy from real estate but lost his fortune in the Great Depression. His childhood was made difficult by his parents' unhappy marriage, which ended when he was nine years old. He lived with his mother in New York and began to write poetry in high school. He graduated early to take classes at Columbia University. He subsequently attended New York University and Harvard, and in 1935 he published his first poetry. Schwartz held teaching positions at Harvard, Bennington, Kenyon, Princeton, and Syracuse. He drank heavily and changed jobs frequently, often abruptly. He was married twice. During his second marriage he was arrested and placed in Bellevue Hospital after a jealous attack on an imagined lover of his wife. This was the first of several psychiatric hospitalizations. After his second divorce he lived the remainder of his life alone in New York City, continuing to write until his death in 1966.

Anne Sexton (1928–1974)
Sexton was born into a wealthy family in Newton, Massachusetts. She spent most of her youth with her great-aunt, attending Rogers Hall preparatory school for girls in Lowell for two years then a finishing school in Boston before eloping at age nineteen with Alfred "Kayo" Sexton II. From 1949 to 1954 Sexton worked various modeling and sales jobs in

New York, Baltimore, and San Francisco. In 1954 the couple returned to Newton, where Sexton had a child and her husband began work for her father's company. In 1954, after the death of her great-aunt, Sexton was hospitalized in Westwood Lodge. In 1955, after the birth of her second child, she was hospitalized again, and yet again in 1956 after a suicide attempt. The following year at age twenty-nine, following the advice of her psychiatrist, she enrolled in a poetry workshop. There she met her lifelong friend, the poet Maxine Kumin, and began writing in earnest. At age thirty-two she published her first book, *To Bedlam and Part Way Back*. Sexton suffered debilitating episodes of depression and increased dependency on alcohol and sleeping pills and was hospitalized several more times. In 1974 Sexton committed suicide by carbon monoxide poisoning at her home in Boston. She had published ten books of poetry in sixteen years and won the Pulitzer Prize in 1967.

William Shakespeare (1564–1616)

Shakespeare was a journeyman actor who may or may not have written a number of reasonably well-regarded plays and sonnets.

Percy Bysshe Shelley (1792–1822)

Born in Sussex to a wealthy family, Shelley was educated at Eton, where he was reputedly reclusive and prone to emotional outbursts, acquiring the nickname "Mad Shelley" among his peers after stabbing a fellow student with a fork. Despite his family's traditional political leanings, Shelley began to develop socialist views early on. In 1810 he enrolled at Oxford, where he met Thomas Jefferson Hogg, with whom he published "The Necessity of Atheism." In 1812 he was expelled from Oxford after denying authorship of the aforementioned. The same year he married Harriet Westbrook, a girl of sixteen. Two years later, after she bore two children, Shelley left her. Subsequently she committed suicide. He married Mary Wollstonecraft Godwin (the future author of *Frankenstein*). Shelley suffered from hypochondria and occasional hallucinations, the latter possibly related to use of laudanum. He lost both of the children he had with Mary, and, soon after being attacked on the street, he and Mary left England for good in 1818. In Italy he became infatuated with a young woman, Emilia Viviani. In 1822 he began a journal called *The Liberal* with the poets George Byron (q.v.) and Leigh Hunt. That same year Shelley drowned when his boat, the *Don Juan*, went down in a storm on the Bay of Lerici.

Christopher Smart (1722–1771)

Smart was born in Kent. He graduated from Pembroke College, Cambridge, in 1743 and became a fellow of the college in 1745. While living at Cambridge he spent substantial time in London writing plays and acting. During this period he also developed a reputation as a free spender and heavy drinker, to the consternation of some of his friends, including the poet Thomas Gray. In 1749 he left Cambridge for full-time life in London. Correspondence from friends around 1750 indicates that obsessive religious practice became evident in Smart. He married in 1752 but continued his lifestyle of profligacy, drinking, and paroxysms of public prayer. In 1756 he lost his steady journalism job after a serious fever, and he was admitted to St. Luke's Hospital for Lunatics in London. He was subsequently moved to Mr. Potter's "Madhouse," a private asylum, and remained institutionalized for the next six years with only one short release. During this time he became estranged from his wife. While institutionalized he wrote a number of his most famous poems including "Hymn to David," "Psalms of David," and "Jubilate Agno." Upon his release Smart published extensively, but he fell back into debt and was sent to debtors' prison in 1765 and again in 1770. He died in 1770 during his incarceration in King's Bench Prison. Notably, there is evidence that some of what are now considered Smart's best poems, such as "Hymn to David," were held back from at least one posthumous publication because they were written while in an asylum and were ascribed to his mental instability.

Carl Wolfe Solomon (1928–)

Solomon was born in the Bronx, New York. He experienced depression at the age of eleven when his father died. He attended City College of New York and left early to join the U.S. Merchant Marines. After extensive travel he returned to New York and at the age of twenty-one committed himself to the New York State Psychiatric Institute, sure of his own insanity. During his stay he met Allen Ginsberg (q.v.); reportedly, Ginsberg overheard Solomon reciting from Dostoyevsky's *The Possessed* and responded on cue, thus beginning their friendship and resulting in Ginsberg dedicating "Howl" to Solomon. When Solomon was released he began working for his uncle, the head of the publishing company Ace Books. Ginsberg asked for Solomon's help in publishing poems by their friends Burroughs and Kerouac, though only Burroughs's work was accepted. It was not until 1996 that Solomon published his own writing.

Anne Stevenson (1933–)

Stevenson was born in Cambridge, England, where her American father had moved to study philosophy after graduating from Yale. The year Stevenson was born the family returned to the United States, where she grew up in a richly academic environment, moving between New Haven, Connecticut, and Cambridge, Massachusetts. She graduated from the University of Michigan, where she won a poetry award. After living in England briefly, she returned to the University of Michigan in 1962 to study poetry with Donald Hall. She moved in 1964 with her second husband to Britain, where she has held a number of teaching positions. In addition to her volumes of poetry, she has published biographies of Sylvia Plath and Elizabeth Bishop (qq.v.).

(John Orley) Allen Tate (1899–1979)

Tate was born in Winchester, Kentucky, where his father's business failure led to family instability and parental divorce. Tate attended private school and in 1916 entered the Cincinnati Conservatory of Music to study violin. He left after a year and in 1918 was accepted to Vanderbilt University. Following a leave of absence to recover from tuberculosis, he received his undergraduate degree in 1923. While at Vanderbilt he became part of a group of writers, including John Crowe Ransom, that in 1922 began publication of the literary magazine *The Fugitive*. After college he moved to New York City and married the writer Caroline Gordon. He was productive as a poet, critic, and editor, and served as mentor to Robert Lowell (q.v.), John Berryman (q.v.), and Randall Jarrell (q.v.). While occasionally returning to the rural South, Tate took jobs at Princeton, the Library of Congress, New York University, and, from 1951 until 1968, the University of Minnesota. In 1950 he converted to Roman Catholicism, though he was subsequently divorced and twice remarried.

Alfred Tennyson (1809–1892)

Tennyson was born to a large family in Somersby, Lincolnshire, and began writing at a very young age. His home life was marked by myriad family difficulties including an abusive, alcoholic father and other family members with epilepsy or addictions; one brother was committed to an asylum. Tennyson studied at Trinity College, Cambridge, and published his first poetry with his brother Charles, at the same time joining the "Apostles," a prestigious literary society led by his close friend Arthur Hallam after whom Tennyson named his first son. Harsh criticism of his poetry and Hallam's untimely death in 1833 were severe stressors, and he began "In Memoriam" as a tribute to Hallam. In the wake of financial stresses in 1840, he sought care at Dr. Matthew Allen's sanitarium. He recovered and published again in 1842 with greater success, marrying and then being named poet laureate in 1850.

Dylan Thomas (1914–1953)

Thomas grew up in Swansea, Wales. His father was a teacher at the Swansea Grammar School, which Thomas attended. Though he did not do well at school, he had been reciting Shakespeare (q.v.) by the time he could walk and was writing poetry from age eight. He left school before graduating and began working for the *South Wales Daily Post* at the age of sixteen. In 1933 the *New English Weekly* printed his first poem. He moved to London, where he became known both for his poetry and for his frequenting of local pubs. He married, and in 1945 a wealthy patron began to support Thomas's work and family, while his marriage suffered from suspicion of affairs. In 1950 Thomas left on his first tour of the United States, where his readings were widely acclaimed. His alcohol use worsened on each tour, until in 1953, staying in New York City for a reading, he died in his hotel room. The exact cause of death is not clear, but several sources provide evidence that it was alcohol-related.

Edward Thomas (1878–1917)

Thomas was born in London. He married and had a child, working as a critic and journalist, and battling depression. His early interest in nature and the environment was stimulated when Robert Frost's family moved in next door and the two became friends. Thomas took Frost's advice and began writing poetry in 1914, initially using the pen name "Edward Eastaway." In 1915 he debated returning with Frost to America, but instead enlisted to fight in World War I. He was killed while serving as a lieutenant in the battle of Arras.

Thomas Traherne (c. 1637–1674)

Traherne was born in Hereford to a shoemaker, yet found the means to attend Oxford. At Brasenose College he began his religious education, and in 1660 he was ordained a priest. In 1669 he received his bachelor of divinity from Oxford, and then moved to London where he worked as a chaplain to Sir Orlando Bridgeman. He became sick and died shortly after Bridgeman died in 1674, having published only one poem. However, a plethora of unpublished religious writing was subsequently discovered. Despite initially being credited to a friend, his work was finally published under his name three hundred years after his death.

Quincy Troupe (1943–)

Troupe was born in New York City and grew up in St. Louis. He attended Grambling College and then moved to Los Angeles and entered Los Angeles City College. His first poem was published in *Paris Match* in 1964. In 1966 he began teaching writing in Los Angeles, heading the Watts Writers Workshop and focusing much of his writing on issues of race. He taught at various institutions, including the University of California at Los Angeles, the University of California at Berkeley, Richmond College, Ohio University, the University of Ghana, City University of New York, California State University, Columbia, and the University of California at San Diego. He wrote for the magazine *Code*, and in 1989 he worked with Miles Davis on the jazz musician's autobiography. He served as the first poet laureate of California in 2002. He lives in La Jolla with his wife and child.

Brian Turner (1967–)

Turner earned an MFA from the University of Oregon and lived in South Korea for a year before serving for seven years in the U.S. Army. He was an infantry team leader for a year in Iraq beginning in November 2003, with the Third Stryker Brigade Combat Team, Second Infantry Division. Prior to that, he was deployed to Bosnia-Herzegovina from 1999 to 2000 with the Tenth Mountain Division. His poetry has been published in *Poetry Daily, The Georgia Review*, and other journals, as well as in *Voices in Wartime*, published in conjunction with the feature-length documentary film of the same name. In 2007 he received an NEA Literature Fellowship in Poetry. In 2005 he won the Beatrice Hawley Award for *Here, Bullet,* from which the selected poem is taken.

Edward Ward (1667–1731)

Little is know of Ward's life. He was most likely born in Leicestershire. It is suspected he received relatively little formal education. By 1691 he was publishing pamphlets in London. He left for Jamaica in 1697 in an attempt to seek his fortune, or perhaps evade his debts, but soon returned to London, subsequently finding an audience for his travel poetry, political satire, and irreverent commentaries on tavern life and the uselessness of marriage.

Thomas Warton (1728–1790)

Warton was born in Basingstoke, Hampshire. He was home-schooled by his father and wrote his first poem when he was nine. He attended Winchester College and then Trinity College, Oxford. In 1747, the same year he graduated from Oxford, he was named poet laureate of the university for two years. He taught poetry there for ten years and became a fellow of Trinity College. He never married. In 1785 he was named poet laureate of England.

Isaac Watts (1674–1748)

Watts was born in Southampton, where his family was subject to intermittent religious persecution. When his father's preparatory school closed and he was arrested, the family moved to London for two years. Watts began to write poetry at the age of eight, and at age sixteen he moved to London and studied at a nonconformist academy in Newington Green. He then began to work as a minister at age twenty-four in Newington, though his work was often hampered by serious illness. Following one of these bouts of illness, Watts was invited by Sir Thomas Abney to recover at his country estate in Hertfordshire. What had been intended as a short stay became a thirty-six-year residence, until Watts's death. During his time at Hertfordshire he continued to write and to commute to London for work when he was able, dying at age seventy-five after several weeks of delirium.

Sir Henry Wotton (1568–1639)

Wotton was born in Boughton, Kent, to a well-respected family. He attended Winchester School and then Oxford, where he became close friends with the poet John Donne. After his graduation he traveled throughout Europe for five years before accepting a position as a secretary to the Earl of Essex in 1595. In 1600 he was hired by the Duke of Tuscany as a spy for James VI of Scotland. He returned to Florence in 1602 and was knighted and named ambassador to Venice by James VI. He remained in Italy from 1604 to 1624, when he returned to England in debt. He was named provost of Eton College and remained in this position until his death fifteen years later.

Franz Wright (1953–)

Wright was born in Vienna, Austria, where his father, the Pulitzer Prize–winning poet James Wright, was studying on a Fulbright scholarship. His parents separated when Wright was eight years old, and Wright subsequently grew up in the Midwest and in California. Wright has spoken and written openly about his psychiatric difficulties and treatment. He works with young children at the Center for Grieving Children and with teenagers at the Edinburg Center for Mental Health. He was awarded the Pulitzer Prize for Poetry in 2003 for his collection *Walking to Martha's Vineyard*, establishing the Wrights as the only father and son pair to win the Pulitzer. He lives in Waltham, Massachusetts, with his wife.

Lady Mary Wroth (1586–c. 1652)

Wroth was born into nobility, the niece of the Countess of Pembroke and the daughter of the Earl of Leicester. She was a member of the court of James I, performing in plays and being married at the age of eighteen to Robert Wroth, the king's purveyor of land for hunting. Her husband shared little of her love of words, while she shared both literary and amorous passions with her first cousin the Earl of Pembroke, with whom she bore two children. Robert Wroth died in 1614, the year their son was born, and her son died two years later. Because of her husband's debts and the death of their male heir, Wroth lost their estate and spent much of the remainder of her life in difficult financial straits. The publication of her long prose-verse work *Urania* caused some scandal as it dealt with themes of romance not thought proper for a woman writer, and which in any event combined characters and events too close to court life for comfort. Little is known of her later life beyond financial records.

Edward Young (1683–1765)

Young was born in Upham, Winchester. His father was a local clergyman and later held the position of dean of Salisbury. Young attended Winchester College and entered New College, Oxford, in 1702 to study law. In 1708 he was named a fellow of All Souls College. He began to publish poetry and plays, and by 1718 his plays were being performed at Drury Lane. In 1728 Young entered the clergy and took a position in the countryside at Hertfordshire. He was married in 1731. His wife's death in 1740 greatly affected Young, though he lived for many more years, dying in Welwyn at age eighty-seven.

Kevin Young (1970–)
Young was born in Lincoln, Nebraska, to parents who had academic careers. He attended school in Kansas before matriculating at Harvard University, where he was mentored by, among others, Seamus Heaney. He spent two years as a Stegner Poetry Fellow at Stanford University and subsequently he received his MFA from Brown University. He has taught at Indiana University and currently works as a curator and professor in the Creative Writing Program at Emory College.

Collections

Popular Songs (published 1801–1827)
The popular songs of the late eighteenth and early nineteenth centuries that are included here are from the earliest published version that could be located.

Poetry of the Insane **(Dr. Charles Mayos, editor; published 1930)**
Mayos was born in Kansas and worked as a physician at both Peoria State Hospital and East Moline State Hospital, Illinois. As a writer himself, he appreciated the poetry his patients wrote and in 1930 gathered the works by asylum residents from across the country for an anthology. The resulting book, *Poetry of the Insane*, contains this poetry along with the author's medical notes about the poets. In his introduction to Mayos's book, Dr. Charles Read's remarks reflect a not uncommon perception at the time: that "mental disorder can make a poet out of a butcher or a banker, by bringing to the surface a previously repressed desire for self expression. And undoubtedly the enforced leisure of institution [*sic*] life may precipitate the exercise of quite mediocre talents." He notes that the quality of the selection is "good, bad, and indifferent" and that the volume is not presented "as a contribution to American verse, but rather as a study of this mode of expression in the insane." Accompanying many of the poems are "Physician's Notes" that comment on one or another clinical aspect of the author's mental state. "The Cure" was written at the New Jersey State Hospital at Greystone Park (no Physician's Notes). "The Awakening" was written at Mendocino State Hospital, Talmage, California (Physician's Notes: the author "shows very little deterioration. . . . Her most prominent symptom seems to be the delusion that people accuse her of being responsible for all the death, disease, and unhappiness of this community"). "The Snow" was written at East Moline State Hospital in East Moline, Illinois (Physician's Notes: "Note the insight in the

last verse, 'My old blue moods—they're always there.' And also in this line: 'Now look what I am and where, please God let me die'").

The Journal of Saint Dympna (Earl "Pete" Nurmi, editor; published 1979)

The *Journal of Saint Dympna* was published for several issues under the aegis of the "North Star Poets" in the greater Minneapolis, Minnesota, area. The second issue carries the subtitle "Writing by the Mentally Ill." This second issue also contains a brief editorial by Nurmi. He writes: "Originally I had planned to print only one issue and then turn the magazine over to whoever wanted it. But the positive feedback from the first issue made me commit myself to the *Journal of St. Dympna* indefinitely. It is a unique project. Mental illness does exist. It has been seriously suggested that it does not. This is incredible nonsense. There are numerous nut theories as to the nature of mental illness. Our contributors can attest to its reality. The brain is an organ of the body like any other organ and it can get sick. . . . Those who submit manuscripts must be, or have been mentally ill. Concerned persons who are not mentally ill must query first." Saint Dympna was a seventh-century Catholic martyr. Legend has it that she was a Celtic or Anglo-Saxon princess whose father fell in love with her. She and her confessor ran away but were discovered in the town of Gheel in present-day Belgium. Both were killed and buried there. In the thirteenth century when their bodies were moved, numerous persons along the route who were suffering from epilepsy or madness were cured, and she became the patron saint of those with mental disorders. Pilgrims seeking cures still travel to her shrine at Gheel. Issue #1 of the *Journal* contains the poems by Lee Merrill and John Appling Sours. The "Contributors Notes" relate that Merrill "writes with humor, a rare quality" and that Sours "evokes too many memories." Issue #2 contains the poem by Mary Coleman; there are no contributor notes for the second issue.

In the Realms of the Unreal: "Insane" Writings (John G. H. Oakes, editor; published 1991)

John Oakes's preface indicates that *Realms* was conceived of as a written complement to "Outsider" visual art. He notes: "We were looking for unusual poems and stories, often by people who had been or were institutionalized. . . . The amount of material produced by these unusual thinkers has greatly diminished in the modern era, principally because of the use of psychiatric drugs that often dull creativity." Kurt Vonnegut, in his introduction, remarks: "Creative people have thoughts unlike those of the general population because they have been culled or feel that they have been culled from that general population. . . . If it turns out that gifted people culled for mental illness have given the world more works of art worth saving then those culled for other reasons, that would make sense, since nobody can feel as steadily and alarmingly excluded from the general population." The authors provided their own brief biographies. Nicol ("By My Own Hand") wrote: "I am a client of the De Nardo Center for the chronically mentally ill. I've lived in Fairbanks, Alaska 9 years." Richard Beard ("The Queen's Foreboding") wrote: "For the past 21 years I've been treated with a number of medications and, it seems, an equal number of labels. Presently I've adjudged schizo-affective, and I willingly attend AA besides—I wound up here in Portland in 1980, climbing off a [G]reyhound, in a mad fury, after over a year of sobriety, to have a few drinks, and I never escaped (It's not a bad city!). I received extensive counseling, and manage to get by. While just another fool for love, I've not been in it for 9 years. Originally I'm a New Hampshirite, attended Syracuse University where I studied with Delmore Schwartz [q.v.], among others."

Credits

The following anonymous poems were used by permission of the John
Hay Library, Brown University: "The Mad Lover" and "Crazy Paul" from
American Mock-Bird; "Song" from *Temple of Harmony*; "Crazy Jane"
and "The Death of Crazy Jane" from *Choice Collection of Admired Songs*;
"Nancy and Gin" from *Boston Musical Miscellany*; "Mary Le More" and
"Away with Melancholy" from *Songster's Companion*; "The Frantic Maid"
from *Songs for Ladies*; "Soliloquy on Smoking" from *The Muse, or The
Flowers of Poetry*; and "Thoughts Suggested on a Thanksgiving Day Passed
at the State Lunatic Asylum, Worcester, Mass., by a Patient."

INDEX OF POETS

INDEX OF TITLES

INDEX OF FIRST LINES